VICTORY Through Breast Cancer

God bless you!
Glenda Sumerel

VICTORY Through Breast Cancer

Glenda B. Sumerel

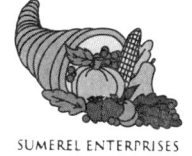

SUMEREL ENTERPRISES

VICTORY **T**hrough **B**reast **C**ancer
Copyright ©1999 by Glenda B. Sumerel

Library of Congress Card Number: 99-93785

ISBN: 0-9671236-0-7

FIRST EDITION
All rights reserved. No portion of this book may be reproduced in any form, except for brief quotations in reviews, without written permission of the author or publisher.

All Scripture quotations are from the Holy Bible, New King James Version, Copyright ©1982 by Thomas Nelson, Inc.

Book Cover Designed by Jostens Graphics

Printed in the United States of America
    By Jostens Graphics

Published by: Sumerel Enterprises
              P.O. Box 905
              Harrisburg, NC 28075-0905

Dedicated to the Glory of God

If anyone speaks, let him speak as the oracles of God. If anyone ministers, let him do it as with the ability which God supplies, that in all things God may be glorified through Christ Jesus, to whom belong the glory and the dominion forever and ever.

Amen.

I Peter 4: 11

Acknowledgments

I would like to thank all of those who have helped make this book possible. First and foremost, I thank God. Without Him, there wouldn't have been a victory or a story to tell.

Loving appreciation goes to my family DeLane, Andrew, and Rebecca, for their love and support during our lives together, during my illness, and throughout the writing of this book. I love all three of you so much, and I praise God for giving you to me to love and nurture.

Many thanks to my parents, Ralph (deceased) and K. D. (Kathleen Dale) Bowling, for the numerous ways you helped me during my illness and throughout my life. Thank you for encouraging me in writing this book. I love you both very much, and I thank God for giving me to you to be your daughter.

I would like to thank my sister, Dale Allison, for her love to me during my bout with cancer, and throughout my life. I love you, Dale, and I pray God's blessings on you, Jim, and April.

Of course, I am grateful to Roger and Linda Byrd for personalizing their license tag with Philippians 4:19. You two are very special, and I pray that God will continue to use you effectively as you minister to others.

My appreciation goes to my church family at Providence Baptist Church in Harrisburg, North Carolina. Thank you for the tremendous outpouring of love and concern for me and my family during the course of my cancer, and throughout the years we have been at Providence.

I also want to thank our neighbors, friends, and relatives for sharing unselfishly with us.

Special thanks to Myra McGarrell and Lynne Allred for proof-reading this book. Thank you both for believing in me, and for your individual parts in getting this book in print.

Finally, thanks to Ed Bohannon for his direction in publishing my book.

Thanks to all of you for impacting my life. I pray that God will richly bless each of you.

In His love,
Glenda B. Sumerel

Contents

	Introduction	11
1.	This Surely Can't Be True	18
2.	The Message	24
3.	Surgery	33
4.	All Your Need, My God Shall Supply	40
5.	No Need to Fret or Fear the Worst	54
6.	God's Promise, Always, He Does Keep	67
7.	Additional Trials	80
8.	Chemotherapy	91
9.	The Dreaded Baldness	112
10.	Radiation	129
11.	Thanksgiving and Joy Cannot Be Concealed	148
	Bibliography	169
	"My God Shall Supply"	170

Introduction

There comes a time in everyone's life when they face a trial which they feel they cannot endure. God promises in I Corinthians 10:13 He will not put on us any more than we can bear. To me, that promise has been shown to be true many times over the years, but never more than when I was forty-five years old and found out I had breast cancer.

In the beginning I was absolutely devastated, because I never dreamed I would develop cancer. I am young. I have a wonderful husband, a fourteen year-old son, and an eleven year-old daughter who need me. I am a nurse who takes care of others who are sick. I don't have time to be sick myself. I've got too much ministering to do to be sick. I didn't want to think of the possibility this tumor might be cancer.

Victory *Through* *Breast* *Cancer*

I had six fibroadenomas removed in the past, and felt very sure this was probably just another fibroid tumor. I suppose this rationalization was a form of denial. It was my way of protecting myself from the devastating possibility I might, indeed, have breast cancer. I remained in denial for eight days.

Then something wonderful happened. Even before the cancer was confirmed by surgery, when it was only suspected, God gave me assurance everything would be alright. The assurance came to me in a most unusual way. Through that event, I had confidence God would again keep his promise, and would not put on me any more than I could bear.

It was in the Recovery Room where I first learned the tumor was cancerous. However, I had a calm about me only God can give. I was not worried. God would see me through all of this. That day, I had no doubts and no fears. My family and friends must have thought I was still in denial to be taking this news of cancer so well. Then again, maybe they thought I hadn't completely recovered from the anesthesia. The truth was, I had the peace of God which surpasses all human understanding.

VICTORY Through Breast Cancer

****

Be anxious for nothing, but in everything by prayer and supplication, with thanksgiving, let your requests be made known to God; and the peace of God, which surpasses all understanding, will guard your hearts and minds through Christ Jesus.
Philippians 4: 6-7

****

That was the reason I was so calm and assured. From then on, I prayed God would get glory from my having cancer. I have been verbally testifying to God's faithfulness and goodness at every opportunity, to anyone who would listen. I can't thank God or praise Him enough for all He has done for me. He has faithfully kept His promise. He did not put on me any more than I was able to bear.

The times I didn't think I would be able to make it past the next hurdle, God was there to lift me up over that obstacle. The times I felt trapped in my fear of the unknown, God had already made a way of escape for me.

Victory Through *Breast* Cancer

****

No temptation has overtaken you except such as is common to man; but God is faithful, who will not allow you to be tempted beyond what you are able, but with the temptation will also make a way of escape, that you may be able to bear it.
I Corinthians 10: 13

****

Willmington's Guide to the Bible explains the biblical doctrine of temptation. One of the definitions of temptation is "to test or prove with the intent of making one stronger". I praise God for how He tested, proved, and strengthened me through this trial.

As we face trials and hardships in our lives, and, indeed, become survivors of those hardships, I believe God wants us to share our experience with others. Just knowing another person has faced a trial and survived it, may help someone who is trying to cope with a similar situation. Maybe that person feels as if his circumstances are hopeless. Maybe he feels there is no way he can win his battle. As we relate the story of our victory over our battle, it may give that individual hope that he, too, can be victorious over his own battle.

I believe God allows us to go through difficult times to make us stronger, in order that we might empower others with courage. My prayer is that this book will empower and encourage you as you read about my.....<u>Victory Through Breast Cancer</u>.

Victory Through Breast Cancer

1

This Surely Can't Be True

Some people have asked if I found the tumor myself, or was it discovered in some other manner. I tell them I did find the tumor myself, but it was only about three weeks before my mammogram was due. It has always been difficult for me to determine if I felt any nodules in my breasts. Because of the six fibroid tumors I had removed in the past, I had subsequent scar tissue formation. In addition, my breasts have always felt rather lumpy. It has been hard to distinguish this lumpiness and scar tissue from true nodules. Therefore, my breast self-examinations have been very sporadic and infrequent.

Because of my history of fibroid tumors, and because I was over forty years of age, I was faithful about having mammograms every year. I also

This Surely Can't Be True

continued to have my yearly physical and PAP smear. Since it was time for my 1995 mammogram, I had already made an appointment to have it done.

About three weeks before it was due, I decided to do one of my infrequent breast self-examinations. To my surprise, there was something there. A round firm mass, about three-fourths of an inch in diameter, and unlike anything I had ever felt in my breasts before. Of course, I was scared and concerned about what this mass might be. Any time I thought about it (which was often), I told myself this was just another of those fibroid tumors. I suppose that was a form of denial. At any rate, it was my mechanism of defense against the terrifying thought this mass might be cancer.

I chastised myself for not having done regular breast self-examinations. A nurse should know better, right? I have talked to other women who don't check their breasts regularly for lumps. That may also be the case for some of you who are reading this book. Let me encourage you to begin examining your breasts monthly for tumors. Early detection results in earlier treatment and a better chance for cure if the tumor is determined to be cancerous.

I called the place where my mammogram was to be done, and informed the receptionist I had found a lump in my breast. She told me to call for an appointment at the Breast Diagnostic Center so that an ultrasound could be done following the mammogram. Waiting has never been very easy for me. Waiting to have this mammogram and ultrasound done, was especially trying.

****

> *My brethren, count it all joy when you fall into various trials, knowing that the testing of your faith produces patience.*
> *James 1: 2-3*

****

Patience is one fruit of the spirit which needs to be more evident in my life. I thank God for helping me to grow spiritually, and for teaching me patience through the trying times.

Finally, the day for the mammogram and ultrasound arrived. The mammogram was done first, and the technician made several different views. I never remembered it taking that long to review the films in years past. I was beginning to be afraid of what the radiologist might be seeing on the films.

This Surely Can't Be True

Eventually, I was taken to the ultrasound room and asked to lie down on the examining table. The lights were low, the conductive gel was warm, the technician was kind, but I was nervous and afraid. It was a fear of the unknown. What would this barrage of tests reveal? Will the tumor look like a fibroid tumor to the radiologist, or not?

I observed the technician for any indication she might be seeing anything profound on the ultrasound. Her non-verbal communication gave nothing away. When the ultrasound was completed, the technician left to get the doctor. It seemed like an eternity before the radiologist came in to offer his interpretation of the mammogram and ultrasound results.

He told me the tumor looked suspicious, and suggested I get a good surgeon and get it removed as soon as possible. I asked if this could be another of those fibroid tumors like I've had in the past. He responded by telling me fibroid tumors are usually round and smooth. This tumor was jagged and irregular in shape and very suspicious-looking. That sure burst my "denial" bubble. I was devastated! This just can't be happening to me! I've got too much living to do yet!

Another waiting period. This time, it was eight days. I asked the opinions of others for the name of a good surgeon. My gynecologist recommended Dr. Peter Turk. Several others had recommended him as well. The earliest appointment I was able to get with him was eight days after the mammogram and ultrasound had been done.

I kept the appointment with Dr. Turk and found him to be extremely nice, somewhat quiet, and very straightforward. He didn't mince words. He reiterated what the radiologist had said about the tumor being jagged, irregular, and very suspicious-looking. He, too, agreed it should be removed as quickly as possible.

We discussed my options. He told me I could go ahead and have a mastectomy to get the tumor out. Or, I could have a lumpectomy with removal of surrounding breast tissue until the margins were clear of tumor cells. He recommended the latter, because he believes women generally do better if some of their own breast tissue can be conserved.

Of course, I know this was just one doctor's opinion. I could have gotten a second opinion, but I didn't feel led to do that. I felt very confident with Dr. Turk's recommendation, and my decision was to have the lumpectomy. He didn't feel the needle biopsy would do any good, because the tumor needed to be extracted whether the biopsy was positive or negative. Thus, my opting for the lumpectomy, would remove the tumor without

This Surely Can't Be True

having to delay the surgery while waiting for the results of the needle biopsy.

He left the room so I could dress, and I started crying. The nurse came over and tried to console me. As I wept, I confessed my disbelief and fears to her. I also told her that even though I was scared, I knew God would see me through all of this. She squeezed my hand and said, "I know God will take care of you, and I want you to know Dr. Turk is a Christian, too." What a comfort it was to me to be assured my surgeon was a Christian.

I left his office in a daze. I couldn't believe all I had heard. I might possibly have breast cancer! What would happen after the surgery? Would I be able to continue working and taking care of my family? My life and the lives of my family would be in a turmoil.

That evening when my husband got home from work, I shared with him all I had been told and my fears. My husband is a very quiet person who doesn't often express his feelings openly. As he held me while I sobbed, I felt his devastation and fears, as well. The surgery was set for October 27, 1995. God had never failed us before, and He would see us through this.

2

The Message

At the time I was going through these tests and hearing this devastating news, I was working the night shift in a nursing home in Charlotte, North Carolina. I had only worked there for about one and a half months. Before that, I had been a critical care nurse for about twenty years. Needless to say, I was burned out with critical care and wanted to try a different kind of nursing. I found long-term care to be very rewarding. The residents were greatly appreciative of the care and kindness shown to them.

I wanted my life to make a difference in the lives of the residents I cared for. I tried to give them hope and comfort in whatever way I could. God also has a precious Bible promise for these dear people.

The Message

****

Even to your old age, I am He, and even to gray hairs, I will carry you! I have made, and I will bear; even I will carry, and will deliver you.
Isaiah 46: 4

****

There was one resident at the nursing home where I worked who told me one night he hadn't seen his family in three years. He expressed to me he surely would like to see them. When I questioned why he hadn't seen them, he told me they didn't know he was in the nursing home. He explained it in the following way.

About three years ago, he and his daughter had a big argument. He confessed he was stubborn, and never tried to contact his daughter or make up with her. So for about a year he didn't see or hear from her. Then he got sick and had to go to the hospital. After that, he was never able to care for himself, and had to be placed in a nursing home. The person who had placed him in the hospital was apparently just a friend and didn't know anything about his family or how to get in touch with them. And the resident had apparently forgotten his daughter's last name. So, the hospital and the nursing home, only knew the friend's name as the person to contact in case of an emergency.

I continued to question him about his family and where they had lived. I asked him to try to remember his daughter's married name. He thought his daughter was divorced and might be remarried, and he couldn't remember the name of her ex-husband. He mentioned several names which he thought her last name had sounded like.

I went home from work that morning and looked in the Charlotte area phone books to try to find the names of his brothers, daughter, or ex-son-in-law. Every town I looked in had none of those names. As I cared for him at night, I often questioned him about the names. I told him I had looked in the phone book for his brothers, daughter, and ex-son-in-law. I asked him to think really hard about what his son-in-law's name had been. One night he gave me two more names that sounded like the last name of his ex-son-in-law.

The next morning when I got off work, I went home and lay down to sleep. Just as I lay down, I thought of this resident and the two names he had related to me. (I believe the Holy Spirit recalled this to my remembrance.) So, I got out of bed, got my trusty, old, phone books and started searching. To my surprise, I found a name which sounded like what he thought his daughter's married name had

The Message

been, and it had his daughter's first name with it. I began to get excited. I wondered if this really could be the resident's daughter.

I called the number, thinking whomever lived there might be at work at that time of morning. A woman answered on the second ring. I explained why I was calling and asked her the name of her father. It was the same as the name of the resident. I couldn't believe it! This was the resident's daughter! My heart began racing. I told her about her dad getting sick and being in the hospital and then having to go to a nursing home. She told me she and his brothers had wondered what had happened to him. She explained to me she had even been looking for his name in the obituaries.

I informed her that her dad said he really wanted to see his family, and gave her the address to the nursing home he was in. She replied that she didn't think she would be able to get over to see him that day. I was disappointed, but I asked if it would be alright with her if I told her father I had talked with her. She said it would be fine. I also asked if I could list her name on his chart as the person to contact in case of an emergency, and give her phone number and address to her dad. She agreed that would be fine, as well.

That night as soon as I got to work, I went to this resident and told him I had talked to his daughter. He stared at me doubtfully and questioned, "Are you sure it was her?" I assured him it was, and gave him her address and phone number.

He gazed at that piece of paper for a minute. Then with tears rolling down his cheeks, he placed his frail hand in mine and shook it. "Thank you," he quietly intoned, "this means a lot to me." I gripped his hand and gave him a hug. As I walked away to begin my shift of work, tears were rolling down my cheeks as well.

His daughter didn't come see him for several weeks. I'm sure there was a lot of history between those two, which I knew nothing about. The resident had to make the first move and call his daughter before she finally came to see him.

****

Let all bitterness, wrath, anger, clamor, and evil speaking be put away from you, with all malice. And be kind to one another, tenderhearted, forgiving one another, even as God in Christ forgave you.
Ephesians 4: 31-32

****

The Message

That is why it is so important to mend our fences at the time they are broken. If we let broken relationships continue, everything is blown out of proportion, and the hurts are so much greater. I was grateful the Lord used me to be a part of that reunion, especially since I recently heard this resident died.

This was just one example of the rewarding things which happened to me as I ministered to the needs of those special people who had given up their homes, their health, and their independence to reside in the nursing home.

Working in the nursing home was an adjustment for me because it was so different from critical care, but the rewards I received made it easier to adjust. It also reassured me I was doing what God had called me to do. Having confidence, that being a nurse was what God had called me to be, made it hard for me to believe I might have cancer. How was I going to still be able to work as a nurse, be a wife and mother, and do all the things I do, if I had cancer?

The day I saw the surgeon and found out the possibility I might have breast cancer, an unusual thing happened to me. It was approximately 10:15 PM and I was on my way to work. As I travelled in one lane, there was a white car in the lane beside me and about a car-length ahead of me. I noticed the license tag read PHI 419. That didn't have any significance for me until I noticed the tiny, little colon between the four and the nineteen.

Personalized license tags have always intrigued me, as did this one. My first thought was, why would anyone write the time 4:19 with the Greek letter PHI. Then it dawned on me scripture is written that way as well. This could be Philippians 4:19. My heart started pounding, and I exclaimed aloud in my car, "Lord, are you trying to give me a message here?" I couldn't wait to see what God wanted to reveal to me.

Retrieving the Bible from my pocketbook at the next stop light, I quickly looked up the verse.

****

And my God shall supply all your need according to His riches in glory by Christ Jesus.
Philippians 4: 19

****

Immediately, I began crying and praising God. I cried tears of joy all the way to work.

Through that license tag and verse, God gave me assurance He would take care of everything.

The Message

While I was sitting at the stop light waiting to turn left, and reading the Bible verse, that car went straight ahead. If I had been even one second ahead of or behind that car, I wouldn't have seen that license tag. I thought to myself, it was just like God to give me a special message and assurance just when I needed it the most.

God knew I would probably worry and be scared when it was confirmed the tumor was cancerous. Through that license tag and verse, He gave me a way to cope with the trials remaining ahead of me. He gave me assurance He would take care of all my needs. I believe the Holy Spirit prompted me to recognize the letters and numbers on that license tag as a scripture reference. As Christians, we need to keep our spiritual eyes and ears open in order to receive all the messages and blessings God has for us.

That night when I got to work, my co-workers inquired about my visit to the surgeon. After informing them the surgeon thought the tumor might be cancerous, I quickly added, "But, let me tell you about the neat thing that happened to me on the way to work tonight." It was just like an old-fashioned revival at work that night as I related the story of that license tag and verse. Everyone was testifying to God's goodness. All were rejoicing with me for having received such a powerful message from God. I thank God not only for the assurance He had given me, but for the person who had personalized his/her license tag with a scripture passage. This happened on October 18, 1995. My surgery was to be on October 27, 1995.

3

Surgery

The surgeon told me he would have to do an axillary node dissection, in addition to the lumpectomy, if the tumor was malignant. All of this depended upon what the frozen section of the tumor revealed. He told me I would be out of work three days if the tumor was benign. However, if the tumor was malignant, and he had to do the axillary node dissection, I would be out of work three weeks.

I had only been at my current job about a month and a half, so, I had no sick time accrued. Any amount of time out of work was going to be without pay.

In addition, the last job I held was at a hospital in Charlotte. I had been there for seven years and I carried my family on the family coverage insurance provided through my employer. My husband was working for a small, private company at the time. Since the company was small, it could not afford to offer insurance to it's few employees. Therefore, when I resigned from the hospital, it was necessary for me and my husband to get some medical coverage insurance.

I knew I would have to be employed in my new job at the nursing home for ninety days before I would be eligible for insurance through the company. My husband and I chose a short-term, major-medical policy to cover that three-month interim period before coverage could begin with my new company. My surgery would be paid for by the short-term policy.

I was very thankful we at least had the short-term policy. We could have opted to take a chance and not have any insurance coverage for that three-month interim period. But my husband and I are not big risk-takers, and we knew too many things could happen to a family of four, even in a short, three months. We also opted not to get the family coverage under COBRA (Consolidated Omnibus Budget Reconciliation Act of 1985) from my previous employer, because the family coverage was going to be entirely too expensive. Therefore, our decision was to get the short-term medical coverage for the whole family.

Surgery

Since I knew I would be out of work for some amount of time without receiving any salary, I wanted to work as long as I could before the surgery. I even chose to work 11:00 PM to 7:00 AM the night before my surgery. One of the day shift nurses came in an hour early, however, so I could leave and get to the hospital in time for my surgery. After leaving work, I went home, got ready, and my husband drove me to the hospital.

I was to have out-patient surgery, with the possibility of staying overnight if it became necessary. My children were out of school that Thursday and Friday. My parents had come for them and had taken them to the lake where my parents live. The grandchildren enjoy spending time with them, and my parents enjoy spending time with the grandchildren, as well. Mom and Dad were going to bring my children to the hospital on Friday morning while I had surgery.

I am so grateful for my parents. Not only did they raise me in a Christian home, but they have always been a support and a help to me during any trial with which I've had to cope.

****

My son, keep your father's command, and do not forsake the law of your mother. Bind them

> *continually upon your heart; tie them around your neck. When you roam they will lead you; when you sleep, they will keep you; and when you awake, they will speak with you.*
> *Proverbs 6: 20-22*

****

My husband, DeLane, and I arrived at the hospital before my parents and children got there. The anesthesiologist teased me about having just gotten off work. He joked that he might not need to use quite as much anesthesia, since I was probably already sleepy.

After I dressed in the hospital gown, the IV (intravenous) was started in the vein in my hand. As soon as the surgeon arrived, I was <u>walked</u> into the Operating Room, and asked to climb up on the Operating Room table. That was the first time I ever had surgery that I wasn't <u>wheeled</u> into the Operating Room on a stretcher. It was a different experience, and one which I liked. I had a sense of having some control over the situation, rather than the situation totally controlling me.

While the surgeon was scrubbing, and the Operating Room nurses and anesthetists were preparing me for surgery, I shared with them about the license tag and verse, and how I had assurance

Surgery

God would see me through all of this. One nurse cried as I related my story. I thank God for the opportunity to share what happened to me, and I give Him praise for His goodness and mercy. There would be many more occasions to share my story in the future.

I awoke that afternoon in the Recovery Room. My husband was with me. Soon, the nurse allowed my children and parents to come in and visit me. They told me David Hix, our youth pastor, had stayed with them all day in the waiting room. Our senior pastor had been with another of our congregation who also had surgery on that day. She was at a different hospital, however. So, David and Dr. Cooper split up and went to separate hospitals. David especially wanted to be there to offer support to my children as I underwent surgery.

I had already shared the story of the license tag and Philippians 4:19 with many of our church family. I was assured there were many people praying for me that day.

With my whole family present, I was told the tumor was cancerous, and that the surgeon did have to remove some of my lymph nodes to be tested for cancer. My thoughts, upon being told, were more of a questioning nature than of fear or despair. After all, God had given me peace through that license tag and verse. I had no doubt He would supply all of my need just as He promised.

****

> *Fear not for I am with you; be not dismayed, for I am your God. I will strengthen you; yes, I will help you; I will uphold you with My righteous right hand.*
> *Isaiah 41: 10*

****

I do remember wondering what was in store for me. Being a nurse prepared me in some ways for the future. But, I had never known anyone closely who had been through radiation therapy or chemotherapy. No matter what was in store for me, I knew God was in control and He would see me through.

Confirmation of that came to me even while I was still in the recovery room. My eleven year-old daughter, Rebecca, had chosen a get well card out of the cards I keep at home. She, DeLane, and my son, Andrew, had all signed the card and had given it to me in the Recovery Room. The get-well verse was on the right-hand side of the card, but the

Surgery

scripture verse was on the left-hand side. It was Philippians 4:19.

I asked my daughter if she had chosen that particular card because it contained that special verse. Rebecca didn't realize the verse was in the card. She had simply selected a card out of the box of get-well cards. My husband and son didn't realize the verse was there, either. They had merely signed the card. I believe God directed Rebecca to the card I needed to see. I again praised God, because He had given me added assurance He would supply all of my need. God is so wonderful and so precious to me!

My surgery had been at 10:30 that morning. By 5:30 PM I was home. My parents had taken the children home with them again, since they knew I would need to rest. My husband took good care of me that night. He had gotten my prescriptions filled, and made sure that I took my medicine as ordered. Later, he fixed a light supper for me. Anytime I awakened during the night, he was right there ministering to my needs. He made a list of all the people who called to check on me while I slept.

The next morning, I read the list of people who had called and I began crying. It felt wonderful to know that so many people cared.

4

All Your Need, My God Shall Supply

That was one thing which helped me cope with cancer as well as I did. The support and encouragement I received from so many people, was overwhelming. I kept a daily journal of what was going on in my life and of my thoughts during the three weeks I was out of work after my surgery. I intended to keep the journal during the process of the cancer treatments, as well. But, after I began working full-time again, I wasn't able to find time to write in the journal. As I read back through my journal in preparation for writing this book, I began to cry anew, remembering all the ways people showed their love and support to me and my family.

All Your Need

The morning after my surgery, my friend, Myra, brought over a meal I was craving. Myra, Yvonne, Priscilla and I all worked in the church library at the time. She also brought a mum from herself, Yvonne, and Priscilla. That same afternoon, DeLane and I were provided with a meal from our Sunday School class. Kathy, Kim, Nancy, and Donna had prepared the meal and brought us another mum when they delivered the meal to us.

The name of our Sunday School class is The Great Expectations Sunday School Class, and our Christian brothers and sisters in the class are wonderful. DeLane and I appreciated the meal and their concern very much. The class constantly lifted us up in prayer, called, sent cards, or just offered an encouraging word to me and DeLane. From time to time, different ones in the class would prepare more food for us. We were and are grateful for the close friendships we have with our fellow class members.

That night, Cindy Long, another of our class members, brought some banana nut bread she had made. And one of our neighbors brought some sourdough bread she had prepared. It was wonderful not having to cook that night. All of our church family and neighbors were wonderful to us during the whole course of this cancer ordeal.

The next morning was Sunday, and Lynne and Randy Allred brought lunch to our house before they went to church. They brought two pans of lasagne, salad, bread, and dessert. Needless to say, we froze one of the pans of lasagne so we would have something to eat another night. That Sunday afternoon, while I slept, Brenda Story brought a huge bowl of homemade chili to the house. By this time, we had enough food to feed us for several days. Mom and Dad brought the children home late that afternoon. It was good to see the children and Mom and Dad again. The children were quiet and helpful around the house, as I continued to rest.

Monday and Tuesday were two of the hardest days of all for me. Monday morning, I called the insurance company with whom DeLane and I had taken out the short-term policy. I knew my policy was only going to last about another six weeks. I wondered what extended benefits, if any, I would have.

Since the cancer had been discovered during the three-month period of our short-term policy, I knew it would not be considered a pre-existing condition. But I wasn't sure if that warranted any extended benefits, or not. They explained that even though the cancer was discovered during the three-month term of my policy and was not considered a pre-existing condition, my extended benefits would

All Your Need

only be for one more month or $1,000 - whichever came first.

I knew in about a month, I would be eligible for insurance through the company for which I now worked. I didn't start worrying until I found out my new company's insurance wouldn't cover <u>any</u> cost for my cancer, since that <u>would</u> be a pre-existing condition. What would I do? How were my husband and I going to pay all of the bills I would incur during the course of my cancer treatments?

Of course, I shouldn't have started worrying. After all, hadn't God assured me He would supply all of my need? God knew I needed a gentle reminder of that fact.

As I was getting really heavy into my worry mode, the doorbell rang. It was one of my neighbors. She related to me the Lord had told her to buy groceries for the Sumerels, and she complied. I know she must have made five or six trips to the car to bring in the abundance of groceries she had bought. Obedience to God brings peace and joy. As she left, with tears in her eyes, she proclaimed, "Oh, my heart is so full!" I hugged her and wept as I surveyed the bounty of groceries she had brought in. My God assured me He would supply all of my need, and He keeps His promises!

VICTORY *Through Breast Cancer*

****

Therefore, do not worry, saying, "What shall we eat?" or "What shall we drink?" or "What shall we wear?" For after all these things the Gentiles seek. For your heavenly Father knows that you need all these things. But seek first the kingdom of God and His righteousness, and all these things shall be added to you.
Matthew 6: 31-33

****

Again that night, some more of our neighbors, the Kisers and the Novobilskis brought a meal over. Another neighbor, Jerry Wallace, brought a cake. Each day God used different people to uphold us during our crisis. And, knowing many people were praying for us, empowered us both spiritually and emotionally.

On Tuesday, I went to see Dr. Turk, my surgeon. He informed me that two of the fourteen lymph nodes he had removed were cancerous. Maybe it shouldn't have been, but that bit of news was quite a shock to me. I never expected <u>any</u> of

All Your Need

my lymph nodes to be positive for cancer. I fully expected the cancer to have been confined to the breast only. I surmised I would possibly receive radiation therapy to the breast, and that would be the end of my treatment. I don't know if this was denial again, or if I had been exercising my faith that God wouldn't put me through any more than the radiation treatments. I wasn't sure how we were going to pay for the radiation therapy, much less the added expense of chemotherapy.

As I explained about my insurance problems and my financial concerns to Dr. Turk and his nurse, I was openly sobbing. Why is it I can trust God to take care of my physical needs, but I act like I can't trust Him to handle my financial needs? Hadn't God given me the assurance He would supply <u>all</u> of my need? I suppose it was because I had no control over what was happening to my physical well-being, but finances was a part of my life over which I <u>did</u> have some control. I had confidence God would allow me to be physically well enough to be able to work and pay bills.

I was in such a miserable state by the time I left Dr. Turk's office, I just had to talk to and be with someone close to me - and soon! My sister, Dale Allison, has her own business, and it just happens to be near Dr. Turk's office. I wept all the way there, and was still crying when I entered her office. Alarmed to see me in such a state, Dale hugged me, then made me sit down and start talking.

I explained about the lymph nodes being positive for cancer, and that I would need chemotherapy as well as radiation therapy. I related to her how worried I was about my insurance and paying future bills.

Dr. Turk had asked me if I could get COBRA insurance through the hospital where I had worked for the past seven years. I had told the hospital that I didn't want COBRA, because it was going to be too expensive to carry the family under COBRA. One COBRA payment for the whole family was going to be more than the monthly mortgage payment on our house. That was why DeLane and I had decided to get the three-month, short-term policy. Dr. Turk advised me to check with the hospital, anyway, because he thought there was a grace period in which you could decide for sure whether or not to carry COBRA insurance.

From my sister's office, I called and found out my time had not expired to make the decision about COBRA. The woman on the phone told me I still had two and one-half weeks to make a decision about COBRA. She explained if I paid the back

All Your Need

payments, it would be as if there had never been a break in my coverage from when I worked at the hospital. I decided to get COBRA coverage for myself only, which would be much less costly than covering the whole family.

When I heard my time had not expired to make that decision, I began bawling and repeating, "Oh, thank You, Jesus! Thank You, Jesus!" Dale came over and embraced me as we wept together. Then she gave me $600 and ordered me to get down to that office and pay those back payments. She reiterated, "I love you, and I just want you to be well."

I did not ask Dale for the $600, she just gave it to me of her own accord. My husband and I had enough money in the bank to pay the back payments, but my sister wanted to do that for me.

Dale gave me that money unconditionally, not expecting anything in return. It reminded me of how God loves us unconditionally. His love for us doesn't depend upon whether we love Him, or serve Him, or are faithful to Him. He just loves us anyway. What a great God He is!

****

In this the love of God was manifested toward us, that God sent His only begotten Son into the world,

that we might live through Him. In this is love, not that we loved God, but that He loved us and sent His Son to be the propitiation for our sins. Beloved, if God so loved us, we ought also to love one another.
I John 4: 9-11

****

I thank God for His love to me, and I thank God for my sister and her act of love, as well.

Again that night, another of our church members, Mary Allen, brought a meal over. After each of these tough days, God used a different person to try to ease our burden.

Dr. Turk had told me I would need to have a bone scan and a liver ultrasound done. Since some of my lymph nodes had been involved, there was a chance the cancer could have spread to another part of my body. These tests were scheduled for a future date. I prayed and asked God not to let there be cancer anywhere else in my body.

On Wednesday, DeLane took me to meet the oncologist. Dr. William Mitchell had been recommended to us. We found him to be very personable and comforting. We liked him a lot. Dr. Mitchell explained about my cancer, the positive lymph nodes, and the standard course of treatment for this type of cancer. Then he described a research study which I might choose to be in, since I met the criteria for the study.

Basically, the criteria for being in the study, was you had to have a malignant tumor with lymph node involvement. You had to be in good health, otherwise, with no active disease, and no metastasis or spread of the disease to any other parts of your body. The study would end when approximately three thousand women had been enrolled in it.

The purpose of the study was to determine dosages of chemotherapy drugs, as well as study the effect and side effects of combining Taxol (paclitaxel) with common treatments for breast cancer. Taxol is a drug which has shown promise in treating some kinds of tumors, and in helping to prevent the recurrence of cancer. Specifically, the study would discover what effect combining Taxol with Cytoxan (cyclophosphamide) and three different doses of Adriamycin (doxorubicin), would have on breast cancer.

In the study, there were six possible treatment arms for which the participants would be randomly selected. A person might receive the <u>standard</u> dose of Adriamycin and the standard dose of Cytoxan with or without Taxol. Or a participant might receive a <u>moderately increased</u> dose of Adriamycin and standard dose of Cytoxan with or without Taxol. Last of all, one could receive a <u>greatly increased</u> dose of Adriamycin and standard dose of Cytoxan with or without Taxol.

Whether I chose to be in the study or not, I would receive the standard dose of Adriamycin and the standard dose of Cytoxan. However, if I decided to be in the study, I might be selected to receive one of the increased doses of Adriamycin and possibly Taxol. Dr. Mitchell explained that receiving the higher doses of Adriamycin and the Taxol, might be beneficial in reducing the risk for recurrence of cancer.

Dr. Mitchell and his nurse told me these were "big daddy" drugs. Some of the usual side effects for these drugs were nausea and vomiting, hair loss, and low blood counts. But there were other side effects to think about, as well. Some of these included cardiovascular compromise with heart rate and rhythm problems, leukemia, anemia and early menopause.

In addition, there was the time factor to consider. If I chose not to be in the study, and decided to receive the standard Adriamycin and standard Cytoxan, only, I would be given one treatment every three weeks for four treatments (about three months). Of course, if I chose to be in

All Your Need

the study, and drew one of the arms to receive the Taxol, my treatment time would be extended. The Taxol would also be given about every three weeks for four treatments. However, Taxol would be given <u>after</u> the Adriamycin and Cytoxan treatments (an additional three months).

Wow! There was so much information to absorb. Dr. Mitchell told me and DeLane to think about it, talk it over, and let him know if I wanted to be in the study, or not. As he prepared to leave me and DeLane that day, he came over to me, smiled and intoned, "Now, give me a hug." Then he went over to my husband, shook his hand vigorously up and down, and instructed, "Now, Boss, you take care of her, you hear." I'm thankful for Dr. Mitchell's special way with us. It helped both me and my husband to relax and feel as comfortable as possible under the circumstances.

When DeLane and I left the office that day, DeLane put his arm around me, sighed, and uttered, "Gosh, Honey, I wish I could go through it for you." I am thankful my husband loves me enough, that he wanted to shoulder that burden for me. We both knew very well he <u>would</u> be going through it <u>with</u> me.

DeLane asked if I was going to participate in the study. I told him my gut feeling was I wanted to be in it. After all, if women in years past had not agreed to be in studies, my treatment regimen might have been a lot tougher than it was going to be. Because of past studies, today's standard treatment for breast cancer has been determined. If my being in the study, could benefit future, breast cancer patients, then I wanted to be in it, even in the face of potential risks and side effects and even if it meant a longer treatment time. Still, DeLane and I would read over the material which had been given to us, pray about it, talk about it, and come to a decision.

****

If any of you lacks wisdom, let him ask of God, who gives to all liberally and without reproach, and it will be given to him.
James 1: 5

****

By the time we got home that night, some more of our neighbors, the Barretts, had brought supper over, and another neighbor, J.B., brought some sweet rolls. Then, David Smith, one of our church members, brought some chili and cornbread his wife, Wanda, had made. We had to freeze the chili, because we had so much food already. I remember very distinctly thinking I could get used

All Your Need

to this not having to cook. Oh, how I praise God for the love and support shown to us during this illness.

5

No Need to Fret or Fear the Worst

On Thursday, November 2, 1995, Mom and Dad came up to take me for the bone scan and liver ultrasound. Dad stayed at the house to answer the phone and take messages, while Mom took me to the hospital. She stayed in the waiting room while I had the tests done.

The liver ultrasound was done first. This felt very much like the time when the ultrasound of my breasts had been done. The atmosphere was similar to that at the other facility. Again, the room was quiet, and the lights were low. The technician was kind and gentle as she cared for me. But, I was apprehensive, just as I had been before. In

No Need to Fret

some ways, I may have been even more apprehensive than when the breast ultrasound had been done, because now I knew for sure cancer had been found in my body, and could have easily travelled elsewhere due to the lymph node involvement. You would think I wouldn't be apprehensive at all, after the assurance God had given me through that license tag and verse. But, we all get into our human modes at times, and that is where I was on that day.

As I had done before, I kept watching the technician for any sign she might be seeing anything suspicious. I couldn't detect anything out of the ordinary in her demeanor. Finally, the ultrasound was completed, and the technician told me she would show the films to the doctor and would be back in a few minutes. Five minutes passed, and she hadn't returned. Then ten minutes, and fifteen. Still, she hadn't returned.

At this point, I was starting to worry. They must have found something suspicious on the films. Lord, what will I do if I have liver cancer?

No sooner had I conjured up that negative thought, than a picture came into my mind. It was an image of God up in Heaven, with His hand on His hip, shaking His head from side to side, scolding, "My Daughter, when are you going to learn to rest in Me?"

The Bible tells us that God chastises those whom He loves. I am thankful for the reproach of my loving heavenly Father at that moment. I, then, confessed my lack of faith, and asked God to forgive me for worrying and doubting.

****

> *My son, do not despise the chastening of the Lord, nor detest his correction; For whom the Lord loves, He corrects, just as a father the son in whom he delights.*
> *Proverbs 3: 11-12*

****

A few minutes after that, the technician came into the room, and happily announced, "The radiologist told me to tell you he doesn't see anything on the ultrasound. Your liver is totally clear." I lay on the examining table and boo-hooed out of pure joy and thanksgiving. The technician hugged me and cried with me.

When I went out to the waiting room and told Mom the good news, we both wept and praised God together. That was the first hurdle that day. Soon, there would be another.

No Need to Fret

The technician called me back to the room where my bone scan would be done. The scan took about forty minutes of lying flat on my back. When the scan was completed, I needed assistance getting into a sitting position, because my back hurt so badly. For several years, I had not been able to lie flat on my back, because it makes my back hurt too much. Of course, back problems is one potential hazard of the nursing profession. I figured lifting and tugging on patients for the twenty-three years I had been a nurse, had probably taken it's toll. At any rate, that was what I had always attributed my back discomfort to.

Having been assisted off the x-ray table, I redressed, and returned to the waiting room while the technicians reviewed the films. Shortly, someone else came and informed me they needed to do a pelvic x-ray.

Here we go again! Why did they need to do a pelvic x-ray? Did they see something suspicious on the bone scan? No! I'm not going to worry about this! Lord, You said for me to rest in You, and that is what I will do!

Mom brought me home and fixed lunch for us. We had bacon, lettuce and tomato sandwiches from the groceries my neighbor had bought for us. After Mom and Dad left to go home, I was walking down the hall to my bedroom in order to change the dressing over my incision. With each step I took, I heard a sloshing noise and wondered what in the world that could be.

Dr. Turk had put a drainage tubing in the incision under my arm where the lymph nodes had been removed. The tubing had been connected to a Jackson - Pratt drain, which is a clear, rubber bulb. When the bulb (which looked like a small hand grenade) became full of fluid from the wound, it would no longer suction, and would have to be emptied. After being emptied, the bulb had to be squeezed flat and the tiny stopper replaced in the emptying port, in order for suction to be maintained. This constant suction, would pull the fluid out of the incision.

When I heard the sloshing sound, I thought the Jackson - Pratt must be full and needed to be emptied. Yet, when I checked the drain, there was minimal drainage in it. I began walking again, and heard the noise again. I soon realized the cavity where the breast tumor had been removed, had filled with fluid. I called Dr. Turk's office, explained my dilemma, and was instructed to come to the office as soon as possible. They assured me they could easily take care of the problem.

I sloshed on over to Dr. Turk's office, where he did a needle aspiration to remove the fluid filling the crater in my breast. I commented that it seemed

No Need to Fret

like he was withdrawing an awful lot of fluid. Suddenly, he teased, "Oops, there goes that full figure!"

"Just how much fluid did you get out of there?" I inquired.

"Enough to change your bra size," Dr. Turk replied.

I chuckled and responded, "Oh well, I guess I'll just have to get one of those Wonder Bras." The nurse remarked that she has a friend who has one of those, and her friend looks great. Then I joked, "Do you suppose the Wonder Bra is anything like those Air Jordan pump up shoes?" We all laughed about that. I left his office in good humor and no longer sloshing.

So what if one breast was slightly smaller than the other. I just praise God I'm alive and well. My husband never seemed to mind having a lop-sided woman. When I finally arrived home that night, it was late. Three more of our neighbors Faith, Martha, and Jean had brought supper over. Later, Shirley, another neighbor, brought me a silk flower arrangement.

On Friday morning, my eleven year-old daughter, Rebecca, got up thirty minutes early so she could wash my hair before she had to go to school. I still was not able to reach up to wash it.

Victory Through *Breast Cancer*

My hair was down to my waist and very thick, which made it heavy and even harder to wash. I had decided I would get my hair cut to just below my ears. As long, thick, and heavy as it was, I assumed it would fall out quickly, as soon as my chemotherapy was begun. I had not had a chance to get it cut, however, and it needed washing very badly. So Rebecca offered to get up early and wash my hair for me. That was so special, having my young daughter wash my hair. I thank God for loving children.

Later that morning, I went to see Dr. Mitchell, my oncologist. The bone scan had shown an area on my lumbar spine which was suspicious-looking. The radiologist where I had the bone scan done, questioned whether this might be an area of metastasis (spread of the cancer). He recommended a CT scan be done of that area in order to rule out bone cancer. Dr. Mitchell, also, feared the cancer had spread to my spine, and agreed with the radiologist we would do the CT scan of that area, followed by a biopsy to confirm or rule out cancer of my lumbar spine.

Dr. Mitchell explained if the cancer had spread to my bone, we may have to do a bone marrow transplant due to the metastasis. He began telling me how factoring in chemotherapy, radiation therapy, and bone marrow transplant would increase my chance of survival and my life expectancy. I told him I'm factoring in God, because with God, all things are possible.

****

But Jesus looked at them and said to them, "With men this is impossible, but with God all things are possible."
Matthew 19: 26

****

Dr. Mitchell agreed God was the most important factor of all. We also decided we would not discuss potential bone marrow transplant any more, unless I had a need to know about it in the future. We would wait to see what the CT scan of my lumbar spine and the biopsy of that area revealed.

I was very tired that day, and took a nap in the afternoon. That night we reheated some of the abundance of food which had been brought over all week. I had not cooked anything since my surgery. That was one part that I enjoyed tremendously.

Not a day passed the whole week, that I didn't have to go see one or two doctors at least once or twice a day. If I wasn't seeing a doctor, I was having scans or tests done.

VICTORY Through Breast Cancer

The weekend was nice, because my family's lives began, somewhat, to return to normal. Rebecca had basketball practice on Saturday morning, and her friend, Kelly, came over after practice. DeLane and I made some banana nut bread using the bananas and other ingredients from the groceries my neighbor had bought for us. I did some laundry, and DeLane returned dishes with thank you notes to neighbors and friends. My husband even helped me shave under my arm and change the dressing over my incision.

Our son, Andrew, helped his dad around the house. Several years ago, my husband began displaying seasonal arrangements in our yard. It began with a Fall scene. The next year, the Fall scene was left up for about a month, at which point, it was altered to become the Thanksgiving scene. Before you knew it he had made a manger scene for Christmas, and finally was setting up displays for Valentine's Day, St. Patrick's Day, Memorial Day, July 4th, and other holidays. We had even begun a tradition of having a live Nativity out in our yard at Christmas time. We would invite neighbors, members of our Sunday School class, and other friends to come and participate in it with us. That has always been fun and meaningful to all of us.

On this particular weekend, DeLane and Andrew set up the Thanksgiving scene. Joan, from

No Need to Fret

church, brought us some homemade chili, to preclude me from having to cook. Some more of our neighbors, the Nashes, came to see me. They were always bringing or sending something over. Rebecca had adopted Mrs. Nash as a grandmother for one of her mission's steps to earn a badge in her mission's group at church. Rebecca and Mrs. Nash got together weekly and prayed and discussed issues of life. Mr. and Mrs. Nash are both very good with many different kinds of crafts. Some days, when Rebecca was there, after their prayer time, Mrs. Nash would help Rebecca make some little something. Mr. and Mrs. Nash would always send me something which they had made. I was so thankful for all of the things they and others did for us.

During the course of the cancer, God used so many people to encourage and uplift us. Sometimes it was someone who called to ask about me. Sometimes a neighbor would see me out in the yard, and come over to ask how things were going. So many people would see me at church and ask about me and the family, and remind me they were still praying for us. I received numerous cards after the surgery, and all during the course of the cancer treatments. The cards always made me cry and were a blessing to my heart.

Myra, the Director of the Church Library, told me many people had come up to her and asked how I was holding up. Sometimes it's hard for us to directly approach a person who's going through a hardship. We don't seem to know what to say in certain situations. I thought Myra gave an appropriate response when she said, "If Glenda laughs, I laugh with her. If she cries, I cry with her."

I frequently received calls from a nurse I used to work with, Gail Simpson. After my surgery, Gail had left some balloons and candy here at the house. That was one of the days we were late getting home, so I missed seeing her. But we sure talked on the phone a lot. Gail is such a hoot! Her quick wit and genuine concern for me, always cheered me.

On Monday Morning, I went to Dr. Turk's office and finally got the Jackson - Pratt drain out. It had been in longer than usual, because I continued to have drainage from the wound. It was beginning to feel like a part of me. I tried to wear loose clothes in order to hide the drain. Even so, it was still difficult to hide the "small hand-grenade" and fourteen inches of tubing. Usually, I just taped it to the dressing that covered my incision.

One day, I was talking to my insurance agent, when the tape came undone. The drain fell out from under my shirt, and just hung there by the tubing. It so startled the insurance agent, that he

No Need to Fret

stood perfectly still and stared at this "thing" hanging in mid-air. I merely picked it up, stuck it in my pocket, and never missed a beat in my conversation with him. After that incident, I always <u>pinned</u> the drain to my bra. I had kept the drain in for ten days, and was glad to be rid of it.

After I returned from getting the drain removed, Virginia Monday from our church brought us some homemade vegetable soup. Later that day, Andrew and I did a little Christmas shopping. That night I went to the Moms in Touch group to which I belong. Moms in Touch is a national organization where moms get together each week to pray for their children and the needs of their children's schools. There is such a great need for prayer for our children.

****

> *"Again I say to you that if two of you agree on earth concerning anything that they ask, it will be done for them by My Father in heaven. For where two or three are gathered together in My name, I am there in the midst of them."*
> *Matthew 18: 19-20*

****

The children of today have to face so much more than we did when I was growing up. There are still too many schools across this nation not represented by a Moms In Touch group. My prayer is that Moms In Touch groups will continue to be raised up all across the country, so <u>all</u> schools and school systems will be bathed in prayer. The Moms In Touch group I belong to, was so supportive of me. Brenda, Connie, Gina, Karen, Mary, Sheila, and Trina especially showed great care and concern for me. Our group has grown to include Kathy and Marsha, and I thank God for those close friendships and the support we continue to derive from each other.

It felt so good to be back at Moms In Touch, and doing some of my normal activities again. The next day would be another milestone in the course of my cancer.

6

God's Promise, Always, He Does Keep

On Tuesday, Mom and Dad came up to take me to the hospital for the CT scan of my lower back. It was rainy, cold, and dreary that morning. Dad asked if I was worried about the scan. "No, Sir," I maintained, "because, I'm resting in the Lord."

The radiologist at this hospital reviewed the scans which had been made at the other hospital, but really thought the area looked more like degenerative arthritis than cancer. He agreed we would do the CT scan of the lumbar spine, and if necessary, we would do the biopsy of that area.

I had to lay on my stomach on the x-ray table for a long time. The technician propped pillows under and around me, and told me to lie perfectly still. I couldn't even move during the breaks in the film-taking. My back was really hurting by the time the scan was completed. Since I still couldn't raise my right arm much, my shoulder was stiff, as well. When the CT scan was finished and had been read by the radiologist, the technician came in and announced the biopsy would not be needed after all. The radiologist determined the area on my lower spine was not cancer, but was, indeed, degenerative arthritis. I went out of the scan room and shared the joyful news with my parents. The three of us embraced, wept, and thanked God I didn't have bone cancer.

That afternoon and evening, I kept "Ma Bell" busy. So many people had been praying for me, and asked me to call them as soon as I found out the results of the CT scan. I never heard so many people praising the Lord for <u>arthritis</u>!

I was still on "cloud nine" when I awoke Wednesday morning. That day I met Dr. Robert Fraser, the radiation oncologist. I liked him a lot, also. The Lord had blessed me with kind, compassionate, knowledgeable doctors. Dr. Fraser explained I would have radiation treatments Monday - Friday for about six weeks. I wouldn't begin the radiation treatments until I finished the chemotherapy treatments. I remember thinking this part is going to be a breeze compared to chemotherapy. I can do this!

God's Promise

Wednesday night at church, I shared the news about the CT scan with those who had not yet heard. Everyone was rejoicing with me that I had arthritis and not bone cancer. After church, I came home and went to bed, because I was very tired. There were many days when I was tired. But, resting gave me renewed strength so I could carry on.

Resting in the Lord, renews our physical, spiritual, and emotional strength. That is why I am thankful God chastised me the day of my liver ultrasound, and asked when I was going to learn to rest in Him. He knew I wouldn't be so weary, if I would just rest in Him.

****

> *He gives power to the weak, and to those who have no might, He increases strength. Even the youths shall faint and be weary, and the young men shall utterly fall; but those who wait on the Lord shall renew their strength; they shall mount up with wings like eagles, they shall run and not be weary, they shall walk and not faint.*
> *Isaiah 40: 29-31*

****

Thursday morning I took the children to school. On the way there, we ran out of gas. I had never had a problem with the gas gauge needle being inaccurate before. This particular morning, it showed I still had gas in the car. The car began spitting and sputtering before we got to the top of the hill. I pleaded, "Lord, please help us get to the service station before I completely run out of gas." The car got slower and slower. The traffic light turned green just as we approached the crest of the hill. I knew if I had to apply my brakes, we would never be able to start going again. Finally, we reached the top of the hill at the same time the car engine died. With the light green, we did not have to apply the brakes, and coasted down the hill to the service station. I filled up with gas, and still got the kids to school before the tardy bell rang. Sometimes, our family-life seems like a sitcom.

I praise God for His care and protection that day and every day. I can't help but compare that particular incident with my cancer. Some days it seemed like I was not going to make it through the day. But, God allowed me to struggle to reach the crest of my dilemma, and then provided the way of escape from it. God is so powerful and so good!

I did more Christmas shopping that day, and saw Dr. Mitchell again. He told me he wanted to start the chemotherapy treatments on Monday,

God's Promise

November 20, 1995. I decided to be in the study Dr. Mitchell had told me about. At least, I would be in the study if it didn't preclude the insurance company from paying my bills. I also decided to have a PortaCath inserted under my skin. This is a small, flat disc which would allow access into my venous system through which the chemotherapy would be administered. I was scheduled to have the PortaCath inserted in out-patient surgery in about a week.

On Friday, I did some more Christmas shopping. I wanted to get as much of the Christmas shopping done as possible before chemotherapy started. Especially, since I had no idea how I would feel afterwards. On Friday night, I did private duty with a patient I had cared for off and on for a couple of years. He is on a respirator in his home. Caring for one person, is not nearly as hard as running yourself ragged trying to care for the patients in the hospital or a nursing home. After I started working five days a week in the nursing home, I was only able to take care of this particular patient every other Friday night from 6:00 PM - 6:00 AM. I enjoyed getting back to work with him. I still had not been released to go back to work in the nursing home yet. There was no heavy lifting or tugging involved in this private duty case, so, I was able to do that kind of work at this point. It felt good to be able to work again.

On Saturday, Rebecca and I went to a beauty salon that sells wigs. I had gone there the day before and tried on lots of wigs until I found one I liked. But, I wanted the approval of my daughter before I bought it. We giggled so much that morning as we tried on wigs of so many styles and colors.

I had chosen a wig with the length of hair just below my shoulders, since I had been used to having long hair. I usually wore my hair pulled back from my face in a bow at the crown of my head. Rebecca suggested, "Mom, maybe you can pull the hair of the wig back in a bow, so it will look more like you." We tried it, and it looked alright that way. In my opinion, nothing looked fantastic. But this one wig looked better than anything I had tried on. Mom and Dad had given me the money to pay for the wig. That was to be my Christmas present from them. The wig had to be left at the salon so Donna McNeely, the beautician who had sold me the wig, could cut it and style it.

After we left the beauty salon, we went to the mall and shopped for a while. Normally, Rebecca can shop until she drops, but I must have worn her out that day. Exasperated, she begged, "Mom, can we please go home now?" We left the mall, ate, and went home.

God's Promise

We had a big storm that evening. Mom and Dad live about an hour away from us in Mt. Gilead. Mom called to say the storm had been very bad at their house. She said a big tree limb broke off, and went through the roof of the house. She and Dad were not hurt, but there was damage to the roof and loft of their house.

****

The Lord is good, a stronghold in the day of trouble; and He knows those who trust in Him.
Nahum 1: 7

****

I was just thankful God protected my parents. Things can be replaced, but not people.

We had a good day of worship on Sunday. Again, many people inquired about me and the family. There were special friends at church who always hugged me, asked how I was doing, and assured me they were praying for me. Knowing these prayer warriors were praying for me meant so much. The encouragement they gave me each time we were at church, always uplifted me spiritually and emotionally.

After church that day, I went to see my sister, Dale, her husband, Jim, and my niece, April. They had recently purchased a Christmas Tree farm, and I wanted to see their new property. My Aunt Inez, Uncle John, and Dad, all met us there. We call my aunt, Aunt Nank. When Dale and I were little, we had a hard time saying Aunt Inez. It somehow came out as Aunt Nank, and that is what we have always called her.

There were two houses on the property my sister and her husband had purchased. The house Dale, Jim, and April would be living in was still occupied by the prior owners. The older farm house had electricity and running water, but it was vacant of furniture. That day, we picked up pecans which had fallen from the huge, old, pecan trees in the yard. We even had a little picnic in the old farm house.

Aunt Nank is a beautician, and I asked if she would please cut my hair. This was quite an event, because my hair had been long for eight or nine years. I kept it trimmed to just above my waist. Some of my family members stood around with their eyes as big as saucers and their mouths gaped open as Aunt Nank cut off a foot of my hair. My brother-in-law, Jim, commented that he could hardly ever remember me having short hair. After cutting off the initial length, Aunt Nank shaped and styled what remained.

God's Promise

It surprised me I did not cry when my hair was cut. I had <u>chosen</u> to get my hair cut, because the length and thickness of it made it very heavy. I thought the heaviness would cause it to pull out faster, as I began chemotherapy. The fact that I had <u>chosen</u> to get my hair cut, gave me a sense of control over the situation. I assumed that to be the reason I didn't cry when Aunt Nank cut my hair.

When my aunt finished my hair, we walked outside to show the others. After the initial length of hair had been removed, the family left to go outside and inspect the property Dale and Jim had bought. Andrew and April had been roaming the land, and didn't even realize I was getting my hair cut.

My son didn't recognize me from a distance, and when we approached them, Andrew did a double-take when he saw me. "Mom," he quizzed. "have you already started wearing your wig?" I explained this was still my own hair, but I had merely had it cut. (Men are so observant, aren't they?!)

Then, Andrew enfolded me into his arms and told me my hair looked nice. Those hugs from my teenage son were so special, because he didn't like to hug as much as when he had been younger.

I wondered how my family and friends would respond to the "new me." I wasn't overly concerned about it, however, because it couldn't be helped. Besides, they would barely be getting used to this new look before I would be sporting another new look (my wig).

When Andrew and I got home that afternoon, I modelled my new hairdo for DeLane and Rebecca. Rebecca never remembered me with anything but long hair. She had seen pictures of me when my hair was short, and always thought I looked "dorky". So, her actual recollection was of Mama with long hair. I could tell she wasn't very excited about my new look.

My husband, who had always liked my hair long, was only a little more enthusiastic about the way I now looked. He did tell me it looked fine, though. I often had a sense that people who told me I looked nice, were just saying that to make me feel good. Many times I didn't feel like I looked all that great, and found it hard to believe anyone else genuinely thought I looked good.

Monday was a full day. I was going to have the PortaCath put in on Tuesday. Therefore, I had to pre-register on Monday. The nurse and anesthesiologist I talked to at the Same-Day Surgery Center, were both people I had worked with at other hospitals in the past. That helped me to relax and not be as nervous about the up-coming surgery.

Sandra Heineken, in the Cancer Center, was going to submit my information for randomization in the study Dr. Mitchell had told me about. Of course, she couldn't submit my information, until I had approval from the insurance company to even be in the study. We thought the insurance company would agree to pay, because these are common drugs that are currently used in breast cancer treatment. The study was more involved with dosages and combinations of drugs, than anything else. If the insurance company granted permission to receive these drugs, then I would be in the study.

In order to be in the study, there were certain tests which had to be done as baselines, to make sure I did not have any active disease in my body other than the breast cancer. I was going to need an electrocardiogram, heart scan, other blood work (in addition to the pre-surgical lab work), as well as my yearly physical and PAP smear.

With baselines established, if any patterns developed in me and the other women who drew the same treatment arm I did, then it could possibly be attributed to the dosage or combination of drugs, for example. Sandra had arranged for the tests and scans to be done on that Monday after I finished with pre-registration. She also scheduled me to be seen by the gynecologist later that afternoon for my yearly physical and PAP smear. Sandra assured me she would continue checking with the insurance company to see if I was approved to be in the study. I left everything in the Lord's hands.

****

Trust in the Lord with all your heart, and lean not on your own understanding; in all your ways acknowledge Him, and He shall direct your paths.
Proverbs 3: 5-6

****

If God wanted me to be in the study, He would open the doors. Of that, I was certain.

On Tuesday morning, I had the PortaCath inserted at the Same-Day Surgery Center. DeLane drove me there at 7:30 AM and stayed with me. I saw two more nurses whom I had worked with at other hospitals in the past. It was very comforting to know familiar people were there taking care of me. Again, God supplied my need for comfort. The PortaCath insertion didn't take long, and DeLane and I left the Same-Day Surgery Center by 11:00 AM. That wasn't bad at all!

God's Promise

I went home and slept the rest of the day. That night I worked with my private duty patient, again. Normally, I only worked with him every other Friday night. But the Tuesday night nurse had needed off, and I was asked to work in her place. I was very thankful God provided me with some private duty work, because I was going to be out of work for three weeks from my regular job in the nursing home. Since I had only been employed at that job for about one and one-half months, I had no sick time accrued. Therefore, any amount of time out of work, would be without pay. The private duty work, brought in a little money to help supplement my husband's income, until I could get back to work full-time. God gave me the strength to work. This was another way in which He supplied my needs. I would need His strength in the days to come.

7

Additional Trials

When I got home from work on Wednesday morning, I took the children to school. That was one nice thing about being out of work for those three weeks. My children much preferred being taken to school than riding the bus. At the nursing home, I worked from 11:00 PM - 7:00 AM. By the time I got off work and drove home, it was too late to take the children to school. However, being out of work for those few weeks allowed me to be able to carry my children to school. My private duty case was from 6:00 PM - 6:00 AM. So, I was still able to get home on that Wednesday morning in time to carry the kids to school. I thoroughly enjoyed the opportunity of doing that for them, and sharing with them as we travelled.

Additional Trials

After dropping Andrew and Rebecca off, I came home and lay down to take a nap. I had worked the night shift for about fifteen years, and tried to minimize interruption of my sleeping time. I removed the phone from my bedroom years ago. I, also, kept the bedroom door closed, so I couldn't hear the kitchen phone ring.

On this Wednesday, however, I kept the bedroom door open. I believe the Holy Spirit caused me to forget to close the door, because it had always been such a habit with me to close the door before lying down for my nap.

****

> *However, when He, the Spirit of truth, has come, He will guide you into all truth; for He will not speak on His own authority, but whatever He hears, He will speak; and He will tell you things to come.*
> *John 16: 13*

****

I had only been in the bed about ten minutes, when the kitchen phone rang. It was my mom telling me she was at the Emergency Room in Albemarle with my dad. She said Daddy had started having pain in his chest, and had said it felt like both of his arms were going to fall off.

Daddy had previously had several mini-strokes in August and September. Then on September 5, 1995, on my sister's birthday, Dad had surgery to clean out the carotid artery in the left side of his neck. The artery had been ninety-five percent blocked, and the surgeon remarked that Dad had been truly blessed not to have had a massive stroke.

Here it was over two months later, and Dad was having chest pain. The electrocardiogram done in the Emergency Room showed Dad was having a heart attack. He was given a clot-buster medicine to try to minimize the damage to his heart muscle. Mom told me the chest pain was decreasing, and they were going to stabilize Daddy, and send him by ambulance to Presbyterian Hospital in Charlotte, which was about an hour's drive from Albemarle.

I phoned my husband at work, and he came home and drove us to Presbyterian Hospital. We arrived after the ambulance had gotten there, but before my mom was able to get there. DeLane and I were allowed to see Dad in the Coronary Care Unit. Daddy was pain-free at the time. But the clot-buster medicine had gotten his blood so thin, that he was bleeding from somewhere, and the doctors were having a hard time identifying the area where the bleeding originated.

Additional Trials

Daddy couldn't seem to stop crying. I'm sure that was his body's reaction to all of the stress he had been under lately. Over the past two and one-half months, he had several mini-strokes, surgery, found out his daughter had cancer, had a hole knocked in the roof of his house, had a heart attack, and was now hemorrhaging. I suppose anyone would cry under those circumstances.

Mom finally arrived at the hospital, and came in to be with Dad for a while. The nurses in the Coronary Care Unit were so nice to allow us to be with Dad as much as possible, especially that first day. We understood, however, they had many things to do for Dad, and we couldn't stay the whole time.

DeLane and I stayed in the waiting room with Mom until about 1:30 PM. I had been up the whole night, and had only slept about ten minutes. Therefore, when we got home, I went straight to bed while DeLane took Andrew to his orthodontist appointment, and Rebecca to her dentist appointment.

Again that night, many people called to see how the minor surgery (PortaCath insertion) had gone the day before. I assured them it had gone well and I was fine. But I asked them to please be in prayer for my dad. Numerous cards came in the mail that day, and every day, which was always a tremendous source of encouragement to me and my family.

Mom spent the night in the CCU waiting room, because she didn't want to leave Daddy. I went over early Thursday morning to see Dad and spend the day with Mom. Mom and Dad's pastor, Nelson Chambers, and one of their church members, Earl Barker, came to see Dad and visit with Mom for a while. They asked how I was doing, also, and I assured them I was doing fine. I, then, shared with them how God had given me assurance through that license tag and verse. I praised God for the good reports from all of my scans. There were many opportunities to share my testimony with others while sitting in that waiting room.

On Friday, I went back to the hospital to wait with Mom. We visited Dad as often as we were allowed. His hemoglobin was still low, and the doctors were reluctant to do the cardiac catheterization yet. Dad still cried readily, and that bothered him. I'm thankful he was able to cry. I believe crying is one way in which we can release the pressure and stress that builds in us. Aren't we fearfully and wonderfully made! I praise You, God, the Creator!

Three days before my chemotherapy was to begin, I was sitting in the waiting room at the

Additional Trials

hospital, when Sandra, from the Cancer Center, called. She was ecstatic! The insurance company had approved payment for the cancer treatments! Sandra had been dealing with the insurance company trying to get pre-therapy authorization. I had told her I couldn't be in the study, if that prevented the insurance company from paying for my treatments.

I was due to begin chemotherapy on Monday, and that particular Friday was the last day in which I could be randomized for the study. I had left it in the Lord's hands, because I wasn't sure if it would be better to be in the study, or not. There had been so many things to consider in making that decision. The side effects and complications. The extended time for treatment if I drew the treatment arm to receive Taxol.

There were advantages and disadvantages to being in the study. From the time Dr. Mitchell first broached the subject, my gut feeling was I wanted to be in the study. I knew I met the criteria, and wanted to do it if it would help other cancer patients in the future. Sandra and Dr. Mitchell told me so few women who do meet the criteria, choose to be in the study. They were both hoping that I would choose to be in it. Besides helping other cancer patients in the future, they felt I would derive benefit from the increased Adriamycin dose and the Taxol, if I were chosen to receive them. At the very minimum, I would get the current standard treatment.

I knew what I personally wanted to do, but what if I developed some of those bad side effects? What would be better for me and my family in the long run? That is why I left it in God's hands. He sees all the way down the road, and we just see the right-now.

Sometimes the answer to our pleas to God is....wait. But, God does answer, and He is always on time. My answer came on the very <u>last day</u> I could possibly be randomized for the study. When Sandra called to say the insurance company had rendered approval for payment, I knew God wanted me to be in the study. I also knew, whatever treatment arm I drew, it would be the treatment God wanted me to have.

Sandra phoned later to inform me I would be receiving the Cytoxan, the <u>moderately</u> increased dose of Adriamycin, and the Taxol. It did not matter I might have more side effects from the increased dose of Adriamycin. It did not matter my treatment time would be extended by three months in order to receive the Taxol. I knew that God was in this, and He would meet my needs as He had promised. I continually praise God for how He worked in my life, and met my needs.

Additional Trials

****

It is good to give thanks to the Lord, and to sing praises to Your name, O Most High; to declare Your lovingkindness in the morning, and Your faithfulness every night.
Psalm 92: 1-2

****

I know when we pray for things, we should expect God to answer our prayers. Therefore, as expectant people, we should not be surprised when He answers. Sometimes, I think the awe and surprise comes in seeing the <u>method</u> God uses to answer our prayers, and in the <u>timing</u> of the answer. Through it all, and above all, we need to praise God for the answers.

Upon leaving the hospital waiting room that afternoon, I went home, cooked supper, and took a nap. That night I went to work at the nursing home for the first time since having had my surgery.

It had been three full weeks since I had worked in the nursing home, and I was glad to get back. Being out of work for those three weeks, and not receiving a salary was hard. Especially, with the accumulation of unexpected bills.

We had to first meet our deductible, before the insurance companies would pay anything. Then in some areas, the insurance would only pay eighty percent of the bill. Our normal bills continued to arrive, and DeLane's salary was the only income we had for three weeks (other than those few nights I had done private duty). Things went well at work that night, but I was late getting off the next morning.

Mom had been staying in the waiting room at the hospital since Dad had been admitted. My sister and I had both offered for her to come spend the nights with us, but she wanted to be close to Daddy in case she was needed. On this particular Saturday morning, she wanted to go home to get some fresh clothes and check on things at the house. Mama was reluctant to leave Daddy, because the day before, they had moved him to a private room. Mom was afraid Dad might need something, and she wouldn't be there to help him. I promised her I would go by the hospital and stay with Dad after I got off work. That reassured Mom enough that she felt comfortable to leave Daddy alone.

Before I went by the hospital that morning, I went by the beauty salon to pick up my wig.

Additional Trials

Donna had ordered it for me, cut it, and styled it. When I arrived at the salon, Donna placed the wig on my head as she taught <u>me</u> how to do it. Next, she cut the bangs a little more, and trimmed the bottom so it would suit my face better. She, also, explained how to care for the wig. After all of the teaching and demonstrations Donna had given me, I felt prepared, but overwhelmed.

I sat in a daze as Donna packed the wig and accessories in a shopping bag for me to take home. Suddenly, I burst into tears. I suppose the reality of it hit me, that I was going to have to be wearing that wig for a long time. Apparently, I wasn't as prepared emotionally or mentally for being bald as I had thought I was. Would I be able to do this?

****

> *Peace I leave with you, My peace I give to you; not as the world gives do I give to you. Let not your heart be troubled, neither let it be afraid.*
> *John 14: 27*

****

By the time I arrived at the hospital, I had myself under control again. I surely didn't want Dad to see me crying, because he would have been upset. I stayed with Dad until about two o'clock in the afternoon. Then I went home and slept until time to go back to work Saturday night.

When I got off work Sunday morning, I stopped by the hospital and saw Mom and Dad for a short time. I didn't go to church that morning, because I was so tired after such a busy, trying week. DeLane and the kids went to church, but I stayed home and slept. I woke up that afternoon to find out the dishwasher had broken. Mom and Dad would later give our whole family a dishwasher for Christmas. My parents have always been wonderful to me and my family, and I thank God for them.

I had a good cry and went back to bed. I slept until time to return to work. I knew the next day was going to be a full day, and I needed as much rest as possible.

8

Chemotherapy

Monday morning, November 20, 1995, was a big day. I had my first chemotherapy treatment. I didn't go by to see Dad and Mom that morning. Instead, I went to Dr. Mitchell's office to receive my treatment. Having just gotten off work, I was a little tired, but they have nice recliners in the doctor's office for the patients to sit in while receiving chemotherapy. Rhonda, the nurse, took my vital signs, and accessed my PortaCath. By this, I mean that she inserted a special (bent) needle through my skin and into the center of the PortaCath "disc". The bent needle had a short tubing attached to it. By using a syringe, the nurse could draw my blood directly through this tubing from the PortaCath. Then it was flushed with normal saline, and IV fluids were begun.

I was given nausea medicine, prior to each treatment, to try to prevent some of the side effects. After that, I was given my first dose of Adriamycin. It was pushed in the tubing over about thirty minutes. Once the Adriamycin had been pushed and the tubing flushed with IV fluids, I received my first dose of Cytoxan. This was followed by more IV fluids.

The whole process took about three hours. My vital signs were checked frequently during the administration of the chemotherapy to ensure that I didn't suffer any adverse reactions from the first treatment. During the administration, I was able to recline in the chair and actually sleep for a while. I don't know what I expected, but, that first day of treatment wasn't bad at all.

I left there, drove home, and took a dose of nausea medicine (again, as a preventive). Needless to say, I slept very well when I finally got home. Ann and Frank Dantism, in our Sunday School class had asked if they could provide us with a meal Monday night, since they knew I would be receiving my first chemotherapy treatment and might not feel like cooking. Of course, I assured them that would be wonderful. The meal was great! I had no problems eating it, and I never got sick that night.

Chemotherapy

I had asked to be off from work on that particular night, since I didn't know how I would feel. I had been scheduled to be off on Wednesday, but they switched me so I could be off on Monday night, instead. Many cards arrived that day, and many people called to see how my first treatment had gone. People constantly assured me they were praying for me and my family, and that was a never-ending source of encouragement for us.

Since I had drawn the treatment arm which had the <u>moderately increased</u> dose of Adriamycin, it had to be administered over two days. The standard dose of Adriamycin could be given over one day, but the dose I was to receive, had to be given over two days. On Tuesday morning, after a good night's sleep, free of nausea or vomiting, I returned to Dr. Mitchell's office to receive the second part of the Adriamycin dose.

The nurses in Dr. Mitchell's office are so nice. Rhonda soon married and moved away. That left Cathy and DeLeslie. They would arrive in the office as early as I needed them to, in order to make it easier for me to receive my treatments. Generally, I stopped by there after I got off work from the night shift to receive my treatment. Usually, I got there around 7:30 AM, but the nurses were always there waiting for me to arrive. I appreciated that convenience so much.

Often, while I was receiving my chemotherapy, Patty, the chaplain in Dr. Mitchell's office, would sit and talk to me. She was always very attentive and supportive. Patty, Cathy, and DeLeslie have all cried with me at times. Even the ancillary staff in the office were great. They seemed to go above and beyond in helping with bill payments, insurance, appointments and anything I had need of. They were all a tremendous emotional support to me.

Since I didn't have to receive the Cytoxan on the second day of treatment, my treatment time was cut in half. "Taxi Mom" left the office that morning to pick Andrew up at school, because he had an 11:00 AM orthodontist appointment.

After returning Andrew to school for the rest of the day, I went to see Dad and Mom at the hospital. Dad was doing much better that day. While I had been having my first chemotherapy the day before, Daddy was having a cardiac catheterization with angioplasty (balloon procedure) to open the blocked artery that had led to his having a heart attack. The hemorrhaging had apparently stopped, and Dad had stabilized enough, that the doctors felt confident he would do fine during the catheterization.

Upon returning home, I fixed supper and took a short nap. Andrew went to a birthday party at a

Chemotherapy

friend's house. Lynn Richardson, from our church, had offered to take Rebecca shopping to give Rebecca a break. That was very sweet of Lynn, and Rebecca and I appreciated it very much. I called to see how Dad was doing. He was doing really well, and Jason and Cindy from their church were visiting at the time. Not only was I receiving support from my circle of friends, but my parents were receiving support from their circle of friends, as well.

****

But do not forget to do good and to share, for with such sacrifices God is well pleased.
Hebrews 13: 16

****

I went to work that night after having received chemotherapy that morning, and did very well. I only had waves of nausea occasionally, and took the nausea pills if I needed them. I didn't know it at the time, but this would be the pattern during the whole course of my treatments. I am so thankful that God precluded me from experiencing any bad side effects.

Carmie Cook, one of our church members, told me that her mom had just started chemotherapy, also. I asked Carmie if I could call her mom and talk with her. Carmie gave me the number, and I phoned. It was great being able to talk to someone else who was experiencing some of the same things I was.

The American Cancer Society sponsors a cancer support program called Reach to Recovery. In this program, specially trained women, who are breast cancer survivors, are connected with women who need information and support during their treatment for breast cancer. These volunteers provide medical advice, emotional support, and information on prosthesis and reconstruction. Reach to Recovery visits and materials are provided free of charge. A follow-up visit can be requested, but long-term support is not the program's objective.

Being able to talk to someone with a similar experience is both exciting and encouraging. That is why I enjoyed talking to Carmie's mom so much. We discovered we each had to have pillows piled all around us to feel comfortable. I had always been one to lie on my side with my arm under my pillow. With the PortaCath in my chest, just below my left shoulder, I couldn't lie on the left side. And my right armpit and arm were numb down to my elbow, because nerves had to be cut to remove

Chemotherapy

the lymph nodes. Thus, it was too uncomfortable to lie on my right side. Carmie's mom said the same thing was true for her. Since we were both having to lie on our backs, it was more comfortable to prop our arms up on pillows. Our husbands each did the propping.

Dr. Mitchell had told me the chemotherapy would cause my white blood cell count to be very low. Therefore, if I continued to work around sick people, I would have to wear a surgical mask the whole time I was at work. That is what I did. I'm sure that my co-workers grew weary of seeing me in that mask, but it helped to protect me from getting an infection.

In addition to protecting me, the mask gave me many opportunities to testify of God's goodness. When people asked why I was wearing that mask, I was able to tell them about the cancer, license tag and verse, and how God had provided for and protected me just like He said He would. Some of the residents cried when I told them about the cancer. I assured them I was fine, because God had richly blessed me and was taking wonderful care of me.

When I got off work Wednesday morning, I stopped by the hospital to see Mom and Dad. Dad was to be discharged that day, the day before

Thanksgiving. After leaving the hospital, I went home and slept for a while. Later, I picked up Andrew from his friend's house, bought some pies and cakes to take to my parent's house for Thanksgiving, and came home and fixed supper.

As a nurse, I have always had to take my turn working on holidays. That was the case on this Thanksgiving Eve. I took another nap before going to work. I was excited, because I knew that in eight more hours, I would be getting off work to begin <u>my</u> holiday. I looked forward to spending this Thanksgiving with my family.

We spent Thanksgiving at my parent's house at the lake. We had so much to be thankful for this year. Dad was home from the hospital, and doing well. We were grateful the strokes and heart attack he had suffered were not massive. And, of course, I had done well with my first chemotherapy treatment.

Mom fixed a wonderful Thanksgiving dinner, and we all ate too much. Having had chemotherapy a few days before, sure didn't prevent me from "pigging out". When Rebecca was younger, she had a hard time remembering the expression "pig out". She always called it "hog down". The whole family "hogged down" that day. I slept about an hour after lunch, and slept a long time after DeLane and I got home from the lake. The kids stayed at the lake with Mom and Dad. I

Chemotherapy

had to go home, however, because I was to return to work on Thanksgiving night.

I had become concerned about some redness that was developing under my right arm where the lymph nodes had been removed. The redness was spreading to my breast, and the area felt warm.

After getting off work on Friday morning, I did some Christmas shopping, and took advantage of some of the after-Thanksgiving sales. I soon returned home to sleep for a while. When I awoke that afternoon, the area under my arm and my right breast were still warm and red. I called Dr. Turks office, and the nurse instructed me to come to the office so I could be seen. She and the doctor were concerned I might have cellulitis in that area, and the doctor started me on an antibiotic. If I wasn't better by Monday, I was to come back to the office again.

Friday night was my night to do private duty. On my way to work, I was almost involved in an accident. As I travelled down a four lane road, with the speed limit 35 miles per hour, I was in the right lane with another car in the left lane, but a few car-lengths ahead of me. Suddenly, that car had to swerve in front of me, because a third car was travelling the wrong way in his lane, and was about to have a head-on collision with his car. The car that swerved in front of me barely missed me, at the same time the other car sped by us in the wrong direction. I watched, helplessly, in my rear view mirror as that car <u>did</u> hit head-on with a truck that was further behind us.

There was a police car heading in that direction, who may have been chasing that car, and I saw him stop at the scene. I was unable to turn around and go back to the scene to offer help, because the traffic was already slowing down and backing up. I did, however, pray for those involved in the accident, and I thanked God for putting that hedge of protection around me, yet again.

****

> *For He shall give His angels charge over you, to keep you in all your ways. In their hands they shall bear you up, lest you dash your foot against a stone.*
> *Psalm 91: 11-12*

****

On Saturday morning, when I got home from work, I went straight to bed. It had been such a full week, and I was very tired and sleepy. DeLane

Chemotherapy

drove to the lake to pick up the children. On the way home, they stopped by Dale and Jim's Christmas Tree farm and bought a live tree. When I awoke later that afternoon, we decorated the tree and had some great family fun.

Sunday was another wonderful day. Friends at church continually asked about us, and encouraged us with their prayers and support. Patsy Sellers, who works in an oncologist's office in Concord, gave me a Partnership for Survival pin. One Sunday, I went up to the alter to pray and was sobbing. Delores, a sweet Christian sister, came forward, knelt with me and prayed. That meant so much to me. So many others in the church never failed to hug me and inquire about me. I am so thankful for my church family.

****

And let us consider one another in order to stir up love and good works, not forsaking the assembling of ourselves together, as is the manner of some, but exhorting one another, and so much the more as you see the day approaching.
Hebrews 10: 24-25

****

I can't even begin to name all of the people that spoke encouraging words to me or lifted me up in prayer. Without the love and support of my family, church family, friends, and neighbors, it would have been so much harder for me and my family to have coped with this trial. I thanked God always for every person who offered a prayer, card, phone call, or word of encouragement on my behalf.

After church, my family and I went out for lunch, then came home and decorated some more for Christmas. I took a nap, and went to work that night. My underarm and breast were so red, warm, and swollen I couldn't even hang my arm loosely at my side. I had to walk around with my arm held away from my body. That tended to cramp my shoulder and neck until they felt stiff. The whole thing was extremely uncomfortable.

Dr. Turk's office was only a couple of miles from the nursing home where I worked. Rather than driving thirty-five to forty minutes home, and turning around and driving back to the office, I decided to wait for the office to open. I sat in the parking lot that Monday morning until someone arrived at the office. As soon as the nurse got there, she allowed me to lie down on the examining table to take a nap until the doctor arrived. I was

Chemotherapy

thankful for that, because I was always sleepiest on my first night back to work after having been off.

The nurse was very concerned the area looked worse. The doctor examined me and determined I had cellulitis in that area. I was told I would have to be admitted to the hospital in order to receive IV antibiotics.

I was terribly distraught at this news. I was afraid if I had to take more time off from work, my status would be changed to part-time. If I were placed on part-time status, I would not be eligible for insurance. I desperately needed this family coverage insurance for my family.

My insurance problems were among the hardest things with which I had to cope during the course of my cancer. But, the doctor explained I could lose the use of my arm if the cellulitis wasn't quickly brought under control with IV antibiotics. I certainly didn't want that to happen, so, what choice did I have?

I tried to reach my husband to inform him I needed to be admitted to the hospital in order to receive the antibiotics in my veins. DeLane was out on a job, and I couldn't reach him. The doctor wanted me to go straight to the hospital, but I said I would have to go home and pack a suitcase first.

Once home, I was finally able to contact my husband, but he wasn't anywhere near the house. It would have taken several more hours for him to come home and take me to the hospital. The doctor had not even wanted <u>me</u> to go home and get clothes packed. So, I knew I couldn't wait several more hours for <u>DeLane</u> to come home and get me back to the hospital.

Therefore, I drove myself to the hospital and admitted myself once I got there. Soon after I got to my room, a nurse came and accessed my PortaCath so they could begin giving me the antibiotics. After that first time in Dr. Mitchell's office when blood had been drawn from the PortaCath, we were never able to get blood from it again. We were able to use it for medication and fluid administration, but we could never again draw blood from it. Occasionally that happens for one reason or another. I thank God the veins in my left arm held up, so the blood could be drawn from there every time.

It had been a long tearful day. I had cried so much in the doctor's office when I was told I would have to be admitted to the hospital, that my eyes were tired and red. Plus, I had been up all night working, and had only had that short nap in the doctor's office. Needless to say, I fell fast asleep.

I stayed in the hospital from Monday until Thursday receiving IV antibiotics. Many of my family and friends called while I was there. Dr.

Chemotherapy

Cooper, our senior pastor, visited me. And of course, my family came to see me, as well.

My Sunday School teacher, Frank Packard, came to see me and brought a love offering from him and his wife Kathy. They wanted to try to defray some of our expenses, especially since it was Christmas time. It has always been easier for me to give than to receive.

****

So let each one give as he purposes in his heart, not grudgingly or of necessity; for God loves a cheerful giver. And God is able to make all grace abound toward you, that you, always having all sufficiency in all things, may have an abundance for every good work.
II Corinthians 9: 7-8

****

But, the Lord was teaching me to receive from others, gracefully. The Holy Spirit impressed upon me that to refuse the gift, would rob Frank and Kathy of their joy in giving. I thank God for the tremendous outpouring of love for me and my family during this time.

VICTORY *Through Breast Cancer*

People I didn't even know, sent cards to encourage me. The regional leader for Moms In Touch in our area, sent me a card. I had never met her, but she shared with me that many in her family had recovered from breast cancer and are doing fine now. I was encouraged to hear stories of other survivors of breast cancer. I hoped sharing my story with so many other people would encourage them. I received cards from people in my parents' church - some I had met before, and some I had never met. Their church and other churches were praying for me.

My mom worked as a hostess in a restaurant in Troy at the time I was going through cancer treatments. Some of the people who worked with her, and some of the restaurant patrons, constantly lifted me and my dad up in prayer. I was always very appreciative of that, because prayer is such a powerful thing.

I knew my Pierce and Bowling relatives, and DeLane's relatives were praying for us. These relatives often sent me cards, and assured me they and their churches were praying for the whole family.

When Dad was in the hospital, I met a minister who was visiting another family in the waiting room. I shared my story with him. I always had a smile on my face as I related the story of the license tag and Philippians 4:19, how God had blessed me

Chemotherapy

and kept me from being sick, and of how I was able to work full time, even while receiving chemotherapy. People could see I was obviously doing well, even in the midst of cancer.

I was told later, this particular minister with whom I had shared my story, used me and my story as the topic of his sermon on the following Sunday morning. God had blessed me in a mighty way, and I couldn't help but share it.

I'm sure there were probably people in that congregation, who, later, shared my story with others. I'm sure there were many people who didn't know me, and whom I didn't know, who heard the story of God's faithfulness to me. I pray that many were uplifted and encouraged as they heard the story. I feel confident there were people from that church, as well, who were constantly lifting me up in prayer as I continued in my bout with cancer.

I remained in the hospital and continued to receive IV antibiotics for three whole days. Finally, the doctor discharged me. I got out of the hospital on Thursday, and drove myself home since my car was still parked there. My white blood cell count was as low as it had ever been, or ever would be. That was when I was the most susceptible to getting infections.

It was good to be home again, and to be with my family. I had to wear the surgical mask around the house, because Rebecca had a cold. Dr. Mitchell had told me if I developed a fever, he was taking me out of work. I planned to do all I could to protect myself from getting sick. As long as I could stay well and work, I could maintain that full-time status. As long as I maintained that full-time status, I would remain eligible for insurance coverage for my family. The short-term insurance for my family would run out about a week after the insurance at my new job kicked in.

So, I wore my mask at home while Rebecca had the cold. I wore it at work. I didn't get in big crowds except at church. And God always protected me, and kept me well.

I fixed supper the night I came home from the hospital. I took a nap after supper and went back to work that night. It didn't matter I had just gotten out of the hospital twelve hours before. I needed to work, and felt like working, so I worked. I found out the next day I had returned to work quickly enough to maintain my full-time status. That was such a relief to me! God never failed to supply our needs.

Once I got back to work, I was able to continue working steadily. On my days off, I had to run errands, catch up on laundry and housework, and go to the doctor's office for check-ups or blood-

Chemotherapy

work. My schedule was so full, I hardly had any free time. I was occasionally overwhelmed by that.

My second treatment was to be on December 11, 1995. I asked my supervisor if I could be off on that day, and she agreed I could. When I stopped by the doctor's office, my blood work was drawn first. Since chemotherapy lowers the blood count, you must have certain parameters before you can receive additional treatments. My blood count that day was too low to receive the chemotherapy. I was so disappointed! Especially, since I had asked for that particular night off. I would have to wait another week, allow my blood to build up, and see if the count was high enough in a week's time for me to receive the second treatment.

I never tried to arrange for nights off on chemotherapy days again, because I was never sure if I would be able to have my treatments, or not.

Finally, December 18, 1995 arrived. It had been four weeks since I had received my first chemotherapy treatment. As I explained before, the nurses had not been able to draw blood from my PortaCath since the first time. They would do fingersticks as often as possible in order to try to save the veins in my arm. My fingerstick bloodwork revealed my counts were <u>still</u> too low to receive chemotherapy. I was told I would have to wait, yet, another week to try to receive my treatment. <u>Disappointed</u> doesn't even begin to describe how I felt!

I was so discouraged, and cried so hard, that Cathy paged Patty, the chaplain, to please come and talk with me. Patty came to the chemotherapy room in Dr. Mitchell's office and talked to me. Actually, she did more listening than talking. She allowed me to ventilate. I left the office in tears, and got as far as the elevators. Suddenly, I felt impressed to go back into the office and ask the nurse to draw the blood from my arm, to see if there was perhaps a difference in the result of the fingerstick blood and the blood drawn directly from my vein.

In their experience, the fingerstick results were always comparable to the PortaCath results, or the results of the blood drawn directly from veins. But to appease me, DeLeslie drew the blood from the vein in my arm. To the surprise of all of us, my counts were much higher than before. I would be able to receive my second treatment that day, after all!

I had prayed all week for my counts to be high enough for me to be able to have the treatment. I felt very confident they would be. Of course, I was upset when the fingerstick blood seemed to indicate my counts were still too low. Maybe, God wanted to see a little demonstration of my faith before he

Chemotherapy

answered my prayer. Whatever the reason, I definitely believe it was the Holy Spirit who prompted me to return to the office to have the blood drawn from the vein in my arm. From that day on, we never did fingersticks again. We always drew the blood directly from my arm.

9

The Dreaded Baldness

My hair had begun shedding excessively by the first week in December. I could run my fingers through it, and the hair would come out in wads. When I got off work the morning of December 6, 1995, I stopped by the beauty salon where I had gotten the wig. Donna, who had sold me the wig wasn't there yet. But Linda, the other beautician who sells and styles wigs for chemotherapy patients, was there.

Weeping, I explained that my hair had begun falling out and was thinning so badly it wouldn't hold shape anymore. I asked Linda if she would please buzz my head. She said she would be glad to. I sobbed the whole time my head was being shaved. I thought I was prepared for this. I certainly didn't cry when Aunt Nank <u>cut</u> my hair.

The Dreaded Baldness

This was an entirely different matter, however. When I had my hair cut, it had been my choice. I had been in control. Having my head shaved was more of a necessity, because my hair was in patches all over my head. This was something over which I had no control.

Linda was very gentle with me, and tried to teach me ways to wear scarves and turbans. I did not have my wig with me, because I had not planned to have my head shaved that morning. Even the scarf that Linda had stylishly placed on my head, did not prevent the tears from streaming down my face as I drove home.

When I got home, I tried putting my wig on and styling it. Not being used to it, the process took what seemed like an eternity. Would I ever get used to this, so that I could get the wig on and styled in a timely manner? I doubted it. I took the wig off and cried myself to sleep.

****

The Lord will perfect that which concerns me; Your mercy, O Lord, endures forever; do not forsake the works of Your hands.
Psalm 138: 8

****

VICTORY *Through Breast Cancer*

By the time the children came home from school that day, I was awake. I hid behind my closed, bedroom door, and asked my children if they wanted to see me without any hair. I tried to prepare them by telling them I looked like a prisoner of war whose head had been shaved.

When I first opened the door, they looked as stunned as I had when I first saw myself in the mirror. But, they both hugged me, and tried to console me. The rest of the day, I wore a turban around the house.

When my husband came home from work that evening, I took the turban off to show him how I looked. DeLane wasn't as surprised or overcome with my baldness as the children and I had been. In that way, he rendered strength to me. At last, we had confronted the anticipated baldness. Another hurdle had been traversed. Now, we could proceed to the next leg of our journey.

I continued to wear the turban around the house for about a week, but it made my head extremely hot. I didn't like it, and gradually wore it less and less. Before we knew it, I was going around the house bald. My husband had been losing the hair on top of his head for the past few years. The kids teased him by saying, "Gosh, Dad, we never thought anyone in the family would have less hair than you. Now, Mom does!" We all chuckled about that.

The Dreaded Baldness

My husband responded by saying, "Yeah, but she is still the prettiest, bald-headed woman I've ever seen." I thought that was so sweet, and that made me cry, again.

A nurse-friend of mine, who had survived breast cancer, told me that having cancer is like being on an emotional roller coaster. I did cry a lot, but it was usually tears of joy. Basically, my attitude remained very positive during my illness.

With practice, it became easier to put the wig on. I wore bows in it for a few weeks, because Rebecca said that looked more like me. Eventually, I quit wearing bows, and just wore the hair down as Donna had styled it.

I did get a short wig to wear when my longer one was being washed, or when anyone came to the door, or when I had to run to the store to pick up some little something. It got to the point where I could put either wig on and style it in less than a minute. I was glad the family didn't mind seeing me go around the house bald, because bald was so much more comfortable than turbans or wigs.

However, the kids were embarrassed for anyone else to see me bald. Anytime the doorbell rang, one of the children would quickly run to the bedroom and get one of the wigs for me to put on.

I had to be careful not to wear the wig while I cooked, because it was made of synthetic fiber. Donna had explained heat would singe or melt the wig. I learned that lesson the hard way.

One day when Dad was grilling outdoors, I reached under the grill to adjust something and apparently leaned my head too close to the grill. Later that night, when I took the wig off, I noticed a patch near the bangs where the heat had melted the hair. Donna had to cut that part out and re-style my bangs. This happened about a week after I had started wearing my wig, and it taught me a good lesson! I never wore my wig near heat again.

The doctor had told me all three of the drugs I would be receiving would cause hair loss. I thought, "that's o. k. So what if I lose my hair....it'll grow back." I was only thinking about the hair on my head. It never occurred to me I would lose the hair on my whole body.

It was kind of nice not having to shave my legs or underarms. I didn't enjoy not having eyebrows or eyelashes, though. I used eyeliner and eyebrow pencil to try to hide the fact I had no eyebrows or eyelashes.

There is a program called Look Good....Feel Better, which is sponsored by the American Cancer Society. I understand it is an excellent program

The Dreaded Baldness

where volunteers offer tips in applying make-up, and wearing scarves, turbans and hats. You are even given a bag of make-up. I never seemed to find the time to go, because I was always so busy working. On my own, however, I tried to devise some ways to enhance my appearance.

In January, 1996, I became very discouraged in my job at the nursing home where I was working. It was a stressful situation for me, and I decided to try to find somewhere else to work. I did not want to go back to the hospital. I had worked in critical care for over twenty years and was really burned out with critical care. I enjoyed long-term care, but the situation at the nursing home where I was employed, was more than I could bear.

I applied at other nursing homes, and accepted a job at a facility closer to my home. It also paid a better salary. I was going to be working the night shift on the sub-acute unit. This was like a step-down Intensive Care Unit, except that it was not nearly as intense as the Intensive Care Unit in the hospital.

I enjoyed it very much. Debra Cunningham, was the Director of the unit, and I had worked with her at a hospital in Charlotte about fifteen years before. I liked the new friends I made there, also. I had been working there about two months when I heard they were going to down-size. Management wanted to decrease the staff on the night shift. This news concerned me, because I was one of the more recent people hired. Based on seniority, I would be one of the first to be laid off.

****

Wait on the Lord; be of good courage, and He shall strengthen your heart; wait, I say, on the Lord!
Psalm 27: 14

****

As it turned out, all of the first shift and part of the second shift on my unit resigned. I was told if I wanted to get forty hours a week, I would need to transfer to the first shift. My salary would not change, so I decided to give it a try. I had worked the night shift for about sixteen years, and I knew this would be quite an adjustment for me.

At the same time I was changing jobs, my husband was changing jobs, as well. We had major changes going on in our lives, but God was faithful and saw us through the adjustment period.

The Dreaded Baldness

It was during this adjustment period I completed the Adriamycin and Cytoxan treatments. If you recall, my second chemotherapy treatment had to be delayed a week, because my white blood cell count was too low to receive the treatment. It so happened that every treatment had to be delayed a week. Instead of getting the Adriamycin and Cytoxan every three weeks as expected, I received it every four weeks. Dr. Mitchell and I supposed the moderately increased dose of the Adriamycin was the reason.

It makes me curious about the other women who received the moderately increased doses of Adriamycin. I wonder if they too had to be delayed a week with each treatment, and received their treatments every four weeks as I did. It's exciting to feel that common bond with other women who were in the same study, and especially those who drew the same treatment arm I did.

I'm also curious about the women who received the greatly increased dose of Adriamycin. I wonder if they suffered really bad side effects, since they received such a larger dose. I know their dose was divided into two days like mine was. And, they automatically received injections to help their white blood cell count replenish itself faster. With these injections, it is possible they were able to receive their treatments every three weeks, but I wonder about the side effects for them.

VICTORY Through Breast Cancer

I am so glad that God made the way for me to be in the study. I feel so good I was able to contribute in some small way toward future breast cancer patients. I also believe I derived benefit from receiving the <u>moderately increased</u> dose of Adriamycin. I fully expect the Taxol to have served to decrease the recurrence of cancer in my body, as well.

Now that I had completed the Adriamycin and Cytoxan, I would wait three weeks before receiving my first Taxol treatment. The Taxol treatments were going to be given in one day instead of two. I would still receive the IV fluids, nausea medicine, and other pre-meds prior to the Taxol administration. The administration process would take five to six hours, every three weeks for four treatments. Cathy and DeLeslie still allowed me to come in early for the treatments. The Taxol treatments started on a Friday, so, every three weeks after that, on Friday, I received Taxol.

Benadryl was one of the pre-meds I received in the IV prior to Adriamycin and Cytoxan. One day when I went for treatment, I sat in the recliner to receive my treatment. Cathy accessed the PortaCath, started my IV fluids, and gave the pre-meds. I was beginning to feel drowsy from the Benadryl, because it was being given straight into my venous system. Also, my words became

The Dreaded Baldness

jumbled, and I asked Cathy, "Does this clair rechine?" Cathy laughed and said, "Oh, yes! That Benadryl is starting to get to you isn't it, Glenda?"

Besides the recliners in the doctor's office, there were rooms set up like hospital rooms. Since, I usually went straight to Dr. Mitchell's office after I got off work, they would put me in one of the rooms set up like a hospital room. That way, I could sleep while I received the Taxol.

I was somewhat apprehensive before receiving the first Taxol treatment. The only problems the nurses had ever encountered with the administration of Taxol was heart rhythm disturbances, and that was only once. Nevertheless, they checked my vital signs frequently with the first treatment to ensure everything remained stable.

I was thankful I never experienced any of the cardiovascular side effects with these treatments. Occasionally, I would have those waves of nausea. But I was still able to work full-time, for which I was grateful.

I did experience a couple of problems after the second Taxol treatment. We still don't know if it was related to the Taxol administration or whether it was just a coincidence. All of a sudden, after eating certain foods, I would have severe pains in my abdomen. Dr. Mitchell thought it might be gallbladder attacks. He gave me some medicine which he felt would relieve some of the symptoms. It seemed to work for a while. Then one day, my abdomen hurt me so badly, that DeLane took me to the Emergency Room at the hospital.

This happened on a weekend. They did bloodwork, and made abdominal x-rays. They considered doing a gallbladder ultrasound that day, but would have had to call in a technician to do it. I asked if we could wait until Monday to have the ultrasound done, because my pain was already subsiding due to the medication the Emergency Room nurse had given me. The doctor consented, and set up the appointment.

On Monday, I returned to the hospital to have the gallbladder ultrasound done. I experienced many of the same feelings I had on the day my liver ultrasound had been done. I remembered the image of God up in Heaven, gently chastising me, and that helped me not to worry as much.

God uses our past experiences so that we have something from which to derive strength or guidance in the future. It reminds me of scripture memorization. Numerous times in my Christian life, the Holy Spirit recalled to my mind scripture passages I had learned over the years. These verses were then used to help me make correct moral decisions, as well as to comfort and assure me in specific situations.

The Dreaded Baldness

****

Your word have I hidden in my heart, that I might not sin against You.
Psalm 119: 11

****

This means we can draw from our memory of God's Word to help us at future times. By the same token, we can utilize the experiences we have hidden in our hearts or minds, and allow them to help us in the future.

Soon, the radiologist came in to talk to me. He questioned me about where the pain had been. He asked me if the pain was still there. I explained to him the pain had not returned. Then he told me he didn't know what had caused the pain. He assured me my gallbladder, kidney, liver, and pancreas were all clear. There was no evidence of stones in the gallbladder, and no trace of cancer anywhere that he could see.

Later that week, I went to see a friend of mine. Evelyn manages Trinity Christian Books, a Christian bookstore out in Matthews. She and I have been friends for about twenty years. While I was there, I saw two other friends, Betty and Arlen Smith. They are pastors of New Covenant Chapel in Matthews. I updated them on all that was going on in my life. I shared about the pain I had been having in my abdomen. I was still having occasional, mild pain there even though the ultrasound had been clear. My friends laid hands on me, and prayed for me.

****

Is anyone among you suffering? Let him pray. Is anyone cheerful? Let him sing psalms. Is anyone among you sick? Let him call for the elders of the church, and let them pray over him, anointing him with oil in the name of the Lord. And the prayer of faith will save the sick, and the Lord will raise him up. And if he has committed sins, he will be forgiven. Confess your trespasses to one another, and pray for one another, that you may be healed. The effective, fervent prayer of a righteous man avails much.
James 5: 13-16

****

The Dreaded Baldness

God honored those prayers, and healed me of those attacks. I never had another attack after that day.

I praise God for His healing. I also praise God for Evelyn, Betty and Arlen. I have known Betty and Arlen even longer than I have known Evelyn. They have offered up many prayers on my behalf over the years, and I am so happy to count them among my friends and prayer partners.

Another problem I encountered was stiffness in my hips, and stiffness when trying to walk. To this day that problem remains. I noticed after I sat in one position for an hour or so, I couldn't straighten completely upon standing. I had to walk a few steps hunched over, before I could straighten my body. After walking those short distances, the stiffness was not as pronounced.

Dr. Mitchell thought it sounded like arthritis, especially since walking seemed to alleviate the stiffness to a large degree. Still, he wanted me to have x-rays made of my hips and pelvis. He just wanted to confirm there was no cancer.

The day I had the x-rays done started out as a normal day. The technician made the x-rays, then came back and said she needed to repeat them. She asked me which hip was giving me the problem. Then she explained the little tag which they have to place on x-rays to show right and left, had been in the way and was blocking a view of one of my hip bones.

That was probably true, but at the time I reasoned, "Why would she have asked me which hip had been bothering me? If the tag had been in the way, the film would have to be repeated anyway. So what difference did it make, which hip was bothering me?"

I began worrying I might have bone cancer, and it was showing up in my hips. After the many lessons God had been trying to teach me, here I was worrying again. Would I never learn?

I immediately left the Radiology Department and walked over to Dr. Mitchell's office. I explained all that had transpired in Radiology, and all the technician had said. It concerned me that I had not had this stiffness two months ago, or even one month ago. Dr. Mitchell told me to go on home and try to stop worrying. He assured me he would get the report, and contact me that afternoon with the results.

Finally, later that afternoon, Dr. Mitchell's office called to confirm that the x-rays showed arthritis in my hips. I'm not crazy about having arthritis at such a young age, but it sure beats the alternative. Of course, DeLane teased, "You might as well face up to the fact you're getting old, Honey." At which

The Dreaded Baldness

point I proceeded to remind him he is a year older than me.

We had received information about Taxol in the beginning. I knew one side effect was it could cause numbness and tingling in the fingers or toes. I was also told it could cause pain in larger joints of the arms and legs. This pain could start two to three days after the medicine was given and last for several days. I wasn't really having pain, just stiffness. Nor did my problem go away after several days. I'm still having the problem today.

I don't know if the Taxol administration had anything to do with it or not. I only know the problem began after I started the Taxol treatments. It is possible the side effect of joint problems could be permanent rather than intermittent as previously thought. It will be interesting to see if other women in the study also developed a persistent joint problem after Taxol administration.

Even though I experienced some side effects from all of the chemotherapy drugs, I am still thankful that God opened the door for me to be in the study. It is very rewarding to know you have contributed in some small way toward the betterment of mankind.

During the whole three months I received Taxol, my blood counts never got so low my treatments had to be delayed. I was able to have the treatments every three weeks as planned. The day I had my last treatment was a happy day! The next day, the florist delivered some balloons and candy from Dr. Mitchell's office. It meant a lot for them to share in my joy of finally being through with treatments.

10

Radiation

I completed all chemotherapy treatments in May, 1996. I had to wait three weeks before I could begin radiation treatments. The last appointment time offered at the Radiation Oncology Department was 4:00 PM. It was already taken. The closest available time, was 3:45 PM, so they scheduled me for that slot.

Since I was now working the day shift, I knew it would be pushing me to get to the appointment on time. My shift at the nursing home ended at 3:00 PM, and by the time I finished report, it was usually 3:15 PM or later, before I could get away. Then, I had to get in traffic and drive over to Carolinas Medical Center where the Radiation Oncology Department was.

There were days when I had an emergency or a late admission at the nursing home, and couldn't get away on time. The folks in the Radiation Oncology Department were always waiting patiently for me when I finally arrived. They continually worked with me to meet my needs.

I remembered asking Dr. Mitchell prior to receiving Taxol, if I could receive radiation treatments at the same time I received the Taxol treatments. I figured this would save me some time. Dr. Mitchell responded, "No, because it would probably rot your skin."

"Oh, o.k!? I believe I'll just wait, thank you! Waiting is good!?!!" (Well, it was worth a try, anyway.)

Radiation treatments were a breeze compared to the chemotherapy treatments. I had to go Monday through Friday for six to seven weeks. I did get very tired during this time, however. I decided it was due as much to having to go Monday through Friday after working all day, as it was to the radiation itself.

Each morning, I would arise, dress for work, and the whole process would be repeated. After the radiation treatments, I had to get in the afternoon work-traffic. By the time I arrived home from the treatments, fixed supper, and ate, I was plumb tuckered out. I would get my pillow and blanket, curl up on the couch, and be fast asleep

Radiation

within an hour. Resting, always renewed my strength.

****

My flesh and my heart fail; but God is the strength of my heart and my portion forever.
Psalm 73: 26

****

That is why the image of God saying to me, "My Daughter, when are you going to learn to rest in Me?" is so important. Resting in God is a safe haven. Also, through resting in God, I was able to have my physical, emotional, and spiritual strength renewed. God really built character in me and taught me so many things during this bout with cancer.

Often, I would pray on the way to work. At other times, I would listen to WRCM (91.9 FM). WRCM is a Christian radio station that plays contemporary Christian music. It has always been a source of encouragement to me. In addition to the music, scripture is read, and prayers are prayed on the air. They have devotionals and preaching. God often used the music and other avenues to speak to me, or bless me in some way. And, yes, to renew my strength. I now support that ministry, because it is totally listener-supported. I want it to keep right on blessing me and others. My prayer is God will also, raise up other people to help support the ministry at WRCM (New Life 91.9 FM). It has truly blessed me.

People continued to render support to us during this time. Cards continued to come. From time to time someone would bring a cake, or bread, or a meal. I really missed not having those daily meals coming in as we did after my surgery. Of course, I didn't expect people to cook for us for ever and ever. But it sure tasted good while it was happening.

We had several family reunions during this time. Mine and DeLane's extended families of aunts, uncles, and cousins, constantly assured us they were praying for us. My immediate family, people I worked with or had worked with, my church family, and friends reminded us they were still praying, as well.

When these people heard my story about the license tag and verse, and heard how well I was doing, they would tell someone else. Then that person would tell another. The "greatest story ever told" spread just like that. One would experience salvation, and share it with another. That one would share it with someone else. Of all the

Radiation

blessings God has given me, I praise Him for salvation most of all. I wrote a poem about salvation, in February, 1990, which I want to include now.

God's Wonderful Love

Have you never heard it said   (John 3:16)
   God loved us and gave us His Son,
So that all who believe on Him
   Will live forever with the Almighty One?

Do you not remember   (Romans 3:23)
   Adam and Eve's sin in the Genesis story?
And because of that, we have all sinned
   And come short of God's glory.

The Word of God tells us   (Romans 6:23)
   Death is the penalty for sin;
But God has provided eternal life through Jesus
   For all who choose to enter in.

There's cause to rejoice and be thankful
   For God's great love for us,   (Romans 5:8)
Because, while we were yet sinners,
   Jesus Christ died for us.

V<small>ICTORY</small> Through Breast Cancer

So, do not worry or despair   (Acts 16:31)
   When thoughts of death, those feelings arouse.
Instead, believe on the Lord Jesus Christ,
   And thou shalt be saved, and thy house.

The Word of God tells us of the road   (Acts 2:21)
   To eternal life Jesus has paved.
And to those who call on the name of the Lord,
   God promises they shall be saved.

So, now that you have heard
   The story of God's wonderful love,
Won't you give your life to Jesus,
   The one who came to Earth from above?

Ψ

   Just as people of old experienced salvation and shared their experience with others, I want to share my experience with you. There is no greater joy than being saved through the death of Jesus Christ, and being assured I have a home in Heaven when I die. I would not be able to live a joyful and peaceful life here on earth without the comfort the Holy Spirit brings to me. I praise God He sent His only son to earth, to die, that I might have eternal life.

   It does concern me that too many people are deceived into thinking they will get to Heaven, when in fact they may not. The only way to get to

Radiation

Heaven is belief in the Lord Jesus Christ as the One who died to save us from our sins and everlasting separation from God. We must recognize we are sinners who are separated from God, repent of our sins, believe on the Lord Jesus Christ, and invite Him into our hearts. That is the only way to get to Heaven. Living a good life, having our name on the church roll, doing good deeds, giving money to church or charities will not get us into Heaven. The only way to get there is through belief in Jesus as the only Son of God and Savior of the world. I wrote a poem about this matter, and I wish to share it with you now.

What Must I Do To Get To Heaven One Day

What must I do
  To get to Heaven one day?
Live a good life
  Some people say.

Give of your money
  To church now and then.
Do good deeds for others,
  And you're sure to get in.

Victory *Through* *Breast* *Cancer*

Get your name on the church roll.
   That's all you need.
Make sure God's commandments
   Forever you heed.

That's NOT the way to get to Heaven,
   One person braved.
Believe on the Lord Jesus Christ,
   And thou shalt be saved.

For God sent His son
   To earth, you see,
To live, die, be buried,
   And rise for you and me.

So, please don't take lightly,
   This gift of God's love,
But be thankful for, and accept
   God's grace from above.

Then the other things will follow
   And fall into line -
Church membership, good deeds,
   Giving of your money and time,

And most of all, telling others
   What you have received,
In hopes that they, too,
   Will repent and believe.

Radiation

My prayer is for you to receive Christ as your Savior if you haven't already done so. Then be sure to share that salvation experience with others. God will honor your testimony, and may use it to lead another lost soul to Christ. As I look back on my life, even before the cancer, I can see how God led me and helped me to grow through all of my experiences. God uses people and experiences to build character in us, and help us in our walk with Him. I thank God for all of the people who have impacted my life. I hope God has and will use me to touch other people's lives, as well.

****

Being confident of this very thing, that He who has begun a good work in you will complete it until the day of Jesus Christ.
Philippians 1: 6

****

I finally finished my radiation treatments in July of 1996. My hair had started growing back even while I was receiving radiation treatments. As my hair started growing more, I wondered what it would look like.

People had said sometimes a cancer patient's hair may came back curly. They said sometimes it would even come back a different color. I always had a little natural curl in my hair, and my hair did come back curlier than before. Prior to chemotherapy, my hair had been salt and pepper gray. I was hoping that it would come back a different color, and it <u>did</u>! Grayer than ever! Hello, Miss Clairol!

It still took months before I felt comfortable enough to stop wearing my wig out in public. It always fascinated me to sit in the Radiation Oncology waiting room and see the hair styles of the women who came there. Some women only required Radiation treatments which did not result in baldness, and had their own natural hair. Others had received chemotherapy with subsequent baldness and wore hats and scarves. Some wore wigs, as I did.

There were two women in particular who intrigued me. One was an African-American woman. She wore big, dangling earrings, very high heels, slim skirts, and was just as bald as I was. There was one big difference in us, however. She was much more self-possessed than I. She was such an attractive, confident woman, the baldness

Radiation

complemented her appearance. I saw her several times, and admired her a lot.

The other woman who intrigued me, was a woman probably in her late forties to early fifties. The one time I saw her, she had on a big-collared, white blouse, full, mid-calf, navy, blue skirt, immaculate make-up, and no wig. She, too, exuded that air of confidence which suited her baldness. I assumed the two people with her were her daughter, and granddaughter. Even they, did not seem discomfited by her appearance.

I never had enough courage to wear my baldness out in public, and my children would have been mortified had I done so. If I ever went outside of the house without my wig, it was purely accidental. That did happen a couple of times, however.

Once, I was going to pick up Rebecca after some school function. Before I was to leave, my husband started talking to me about something. I was concentrating on what he was saying as I dressed. He was still talking to me as I opened the door and stepped out on the porch. Thankfully, my husband inquired, "Well, Honey, aren't you going to wear your wig?" I reached up felt my bald head and started giggling. DeLane and I both had a hearty laugh about that. If I had gotten all the way to school without my wig, Rebecca would have disowned me.

On another occasion, Andrew and I went outside to do some yard work. I got all the way up to the busy road at the corner of our property before I realized that I wasn't wearing my wig. Andrew had followed me out the door, and he hadn't even noticed. Chagrined, I said, "Oh, no! I forgot my wig." Andrew who was further back from me, started motioning for me to get in the house quickly. He even said, "Mom, hurry up and get in the house!" I replied, "No, I'll just stand behind this tree while you bring my wig to me." The tree was short, and leafy, and hid my head pretty well.

I believe Andrew would have set a track record that day as he raced into the house to get my wig and bring it to me. But, I can't complain about my children's embarrassment, too much. Obviously, I was just as humiliated, or I wouldn't have been hiding behind that full-figured tree. I admire any woman who is confident and assured enough to go bald as those two women did. They really were attractive ladies.

It has been almost a year, now, since my hair started growing back, and I'm still trying to get used to short hair. As I pass by mirrors, I have to do double-takes to see who that strange woman is. At church, I pass people and say, "Hello." They

Radiation

automatically reply, "Hello." Then a few seconds later, surprised, they add, "Oh! Hi, Glenda! I didn't recognize you." If I had wanted to be incognito for some reason, I probably could have been.

When I had first gotten the wig, Rebecca had drawn a face on the Styrofoam head that held my wig when I wasn't wearing it. She did that to try to cheer me. I was thrilled when I was finally able to pack that wig and Styrofoam head in a box, and place it in the top of my closet. I was beginning to get some control back over my life!

The thing that finally encouraged me to quit wearing my wig was, I changed jobs again. In all of my twenty four years of being a nurse, I had never changed jobs as frequently as I did during the year after I left the hospital.

The circumstances in the second nursing home, became unbearable for me. The management continued to down-size. They even took away the sub-acute status, and made the unit a Medicare unit. I was working under so much stress I decided to resign. I know stress contributes to cancer, and I didn't want to get cancer again, if I could help it.

I took another job, at yet another nursing home. I would again be working on a sub-acute unit. I was hoping this would be the place from which I would retire. The people at this new facility, had never seen me in short hair or a wig, so I decided it was finally time to pack the wig away. They would probably assume I like to wear my hair very short.

My first day in orientation, I heard that the company was down-sizing. I couldn't believe it! This down-sizing business seemed to be following me around. I know that nursing homes are trying to conserve costs, as are all businesses. But there was the same amount of work to be done by fewer people. The down-sizing directly affected the other shifts on my unit, and the other units on my shift. In those ways, it indirectly affected me.

I had only been at this third nursing home about a month. I was still in that probationary period where the company could decide if they wanted to continue employing me, or I could decide if I wanted to continue my employment with them. I decided it was too stressful for me, so I resigned from there, as well. That was when I started doing private duty full-time.

There are advantages and disadvantages to doing private duty, however. One disadvantage is I am not guaranteed any work. Most of the work I have gotten has been when one of the regular nurses on a case wanted off. Also, a lot of the cases are paid by Medicare. Most cases do not require a Registered Nurse. Medicare will pay for a licensed person, but it doesn't necessarily have to be a Registered Nurse. So, even though I am a

Radiation

Registered Nurse, I receive the same pay as the Licensed Practical Nurses. This caused a considerable cut in pay for me, because I received a good salary from the last two nursing homes in which I worked. On a few rare occasions since I began doing private duty, I received a Registered Nurse's pay, but not often.

I have been doing private duty about five months, now. Meeting our bills has been difficult at times, since I took such a big cut in pay. My parents have helped us financially in so many ways. My Dad's best help was to tell me to get rid of those credit cards, and to try to help me in planning a budget. I haven't heeded all of the advice Dad has given, but some of it soaked in. At least I don't carry my major credit card anymore. The kids know we are having to cut back on our spending, and they are trying to cut corners in every way they can, too.

As I said before, finances was one of our worst hardships during the course of my cancer. DeLane and I had always spent a couple of thousand dollars each summer for a week's vacation. The summer before I found out I had cancer, we had viewed a timeshare location in Virginia. We decided to get it, because we felt it would be a good investment.

With a timeshare, we would have a place to stay every summer. In a few years, the money we would have spent toward our yearly vacations would have been invested in the timeshare. The timeshare we bought, has an upstairs with a partial kitchen, and a downstairs with a full kitchen. So, the upstairs and the downstairs could really be used as two separate units. We would even get a deed for it, and could will it to our children.

DeLane and I had some money in savings, and decided to go ahead and pay for the whole timeshare rather than financing it. Doing so, took a big chunk out of our savings, but we felt it was a good investment. Then, wouldn't you know it, a couple of months later I found out I had cancer.

I thank God He kept me well enough to keep working. One of the members of the church approached me and asked if there was anything special we needed help with. He explained some of the deacons had expressed interest in helping us financially. I told him we were doing alright at that point, but if anything happened to keep me out of work in the future, we may need help then. I thanked him, and assured him I would let him know if we needed financial assistance in the future.

Not long after that, I received some information in the mail from my previous employer. I was

Radiation

informed that as a former employee of the company with greater than five years of service, I was vested in their pension plan. They explained I could opt to take the money as a <u>lump sum cashout</u> or as a <u>deferred straight life annuity</u>. I opted for the <u>lump sum cashout</u>. They sent a check to the Internal Revenue Service as income tax withholding to be credited against our taxes. A check for the remaining eighty percent, was sent directly to me. I tithed ten percent of it to my church, put some of it back into our savings account, and used the rest of it to pay bills which had accumulated.

****

> *"Bring all the tithes into the storehouse, that there may be food in My house, and try Me now in this,"* says the Lord of hosts, *"if I will not open up for you the windows of heaven and pour out for you such blessing that there will not be room enough to receive it."*
> *Malachi 3: 10*

****

God did as He promised, and supplied every need we had. It's amazing to me to look back and see all the ways in which He kept that promise. I praise Him for providing for our needs.

I had forgotten I was even in the pension plan, because the last few years I had been employed with that company, I only worked on the weekends, and was considered as a part-time employee. Part-time employees had no benefits, other than being able to purchase insurance through the company. I had forgotten that the time I spent as a full-time employee had gone toward a pension plan. I could have rolled this into an IRA (Individual Retirement Account), but we needed the money more to pay bills at that particular time. Besides, I already had a good IRA started. God always provided for our needs just like He promised He would.

That is why I am not worried about paying our bills now. We have cut back, and aren't spending for things like we used to. But, God knows what we have need of, and I know He will provide. At least I am not under work stress, anymore, and I praise Him for that.

I am thoroughly enjoying doing private duty. I am still taking care of the man I have taken care of all along. I have cared for other adults and young people with various medical problems. The families of these clients are so nice. The other nurses I work with have all been nice and

Radiation

supportive as I shared my story with them. I can't thank God enough for His goodness and His mercy.

11

Thanksgiving and Joy Cannot Be Concealed

I completed all of my treatments in late July of 1996. By this time, my family and I were ready for a vacation. We traded our timeshare week at Williamsburg, Virginia for a week on the Gulf Coast of Florida. We had a wonderful time. I didn't wear my wig very much while there. Mostly, I just wore a baseball cap. My hair was only about a half of an inch all over my head. It felt so good to be free of that hot wig for a while.

It was beautiful down in Florida. We had so much fun fishing, swimming, and simply relaxing. The resort where we stayed, had a hot dog cookout for the guests on Tuesday. With a dollar ticket, you could eat all of the hot dogs you wanted. The ticket stubs were entered in a drawing for prizes to be

Thanksgiving and Joy

given away. We bought four tickets for our family, and won three prizes from the four tickets. One of the prizes was a free parasail ride.

I had never even entertained the thought of going parasailing, until then. We made a reservation to go on Saturday before we were to leave Florida on Sunday. Of course, we bought enough tickets for the whole family, because we couldn't agree on who would get the free ride.

Andrew and Rebecca went first, and rode side by side. Next, DeLane went alone. The kids and I tried to get the guys to dunk DeLane in the ocean when they were reeling him back to the boat, but they wouldn't do it. Finally, it was my turn. It was a tremendous thrill to be sailing approximately four to five hundred feet in the air. It was really quite calm at that height, and I couldn't help but be awed by God's creation, and by the Creator.

Parasailing was one of the highlights of our vacation. The other one came as we were leaving Florida on Sunday. We stopped by one of the public fishing places DeLane and I had found. It was our favorite fishing spot. As we were standing on shore, and looking out over the channel, we witnessed a mother and baby manatee in the wild. They were feeding on the vegetation at the bottom of the channel near the shore. They swam within fifteen to twenty feet of us. That was exhilarating!

And again, I was awed by God's creation, and by the Creator.

We returned home late that night, and the children returned to school within a week. We don't usually plan our vacations so close to the start of school. However, I wasn't sure if I would be through with radiation treatments in time to take a vacation that summer. In making the reservations for the resort, I allowed two weeks after my anticipated end date for therapy. I wanted a little lead-way in case radiation treatments had to be delayed for some reason.

But the treatments ended on time, and I used those two weeks to pack for our vacation. What a wonderful time we had! This was another time of rest, in which mine and my family's strength could be renewed. It had been a long ten months. With the children starting back to school, our lives were returning to some form of normalcy. For that, I was grateful. I looked forward to not having to go to a doctor's office or therapy on a daily basis.

For the first year after my treatments ended, I was examined by the oncologist every three months. Blood work was drawn at those times, also. I had a chest x-ray every six months. I still had my yearly mammogram. And of course, I continued having my yearly physical and PAP smear by the gynecologist.

Thanksgiving and Joy

My mammogram was scheduled to be repeated in November of 1996. My first three-month check-up was in November, also. I had bloodwork drawn at that three-month visit. It was normal except that my cholesterol was high. My cholesterol was approaching high even before I began chemotherapy. It got higher during the chemotherapy. And was still high in the Spring, when I was receiving radiation treatments. Otherwise, my bloodwork was normal, and this three-month examination did not reveal any problems.

I was somewhat apprehensive about those first check-ups and tests. I suppose I tended to allow my humanness to take charge of my thoughts from time to time. I wanted to believe God would not allow me to have cancer again. But waiting to have it confirmed by tests and examinations, was very trying for me.

I was so excited and happy when I got the report that my mammogram and PAP smear were normal. Of course, my support group was rejoicing with me. I praise God He healed me of cancer, and I pray for it never to return!

Since there is a history of skin cancer in my family, I wanted the dermatologist to examine me to make sure I didn't have skin cancer. I have a lot of moles on my body, and some of them look suspicious to me. But, I wasn't sure, and I wanted an expert to determine if any of them were skin cancers.

Someone recommended I go to Dr. Kerry Shafran in Charlotte. He didn't look old enough to be a doctor. But, I found him to be very nice and knowledgeable. The people that work in his office were also nice.

Dr. Shafran removed some tissue on the side of my nose, and sent it to be tested. It was a basal cell carcinoma. All of it had been removed at the time of the biopsy, so there was no further treatment required. Dr. Shafran did not feel there were any other areas of skin cancer. There are some of my moles that we will be observing over the years, but he didn't feel anything else looked cancerous at this time.

Suddenly, last month, a crusty mole appeared on my leg. I made an appointment with Dr. Shafran to have it checked and removed if necessary. He told me that it was essentially just an old-age spot. It was removed and that was the end of that. Of course, my husband wouldn't let me live that down.

My deductible for my COBRA insurance had been met for 1996. For that reason, I wanted to have as many medical needs as possible fulfilled before the new year began. In 1997, I would have to meet a new deductible before the insurance company would pay any of my medical bills.

Thanksgiving and Joy

As soon as I learned all of my labwork and tests were normal, I decided to have the PortaCath removed. It had been in for over a year, and was no longer needed, and I wanted it out. The surgery was scheduled for December 31, 1996. There's nothing like waiting until the last minute is there?! At least the surgery would be done in the year when my insurance deductible had already been met. The PortaCath was removed without problems. I felt like I was really making progress now!

DeLane and I were both settled in our jobs by this time. It was totally unlike us to change jobs so frequently. When disbelieving family and friends questioned, "You're changing jobs again?", I joked that DeLane and I were just trying to find our niche.

Seriously, we were not job hoppers. My husband had worked at one of his jobs for fourteen years when the company closed, and he was without work. Before I travelled the nursing home circuit, the last three jobs I held, had been for no less than six or seven years each. I was happy that we had each finally found what we wanted to do. My husband was forty-seven years old at the time and I was forty-six. We each needed to settle into a job, and soon. Of course, I was changing jobs more often than my husband. It is so nice not to be working under stress. I feel like a huge burden has been lifted off me, now that I am not working in the nursing homes, anymore.

I do believe God had a purpose in placing me in those three different nursing homes during that year's time, however. I prayed He would make me a blessing to others with whom I came into contact. I believe God honored my prayer, and did use me to minister to the needs of those in the nursing homes. Many of the residents and staff blessed me in return. I thank God for my experiences during that year. I believe God used the hard, stressful times to make me appreciate the not-stressful times now.

I try to look at tough times as character-building times, and I praise God for them.

****

> *And not only that, but we also glory in tribulations, knowing that tribulation produces perseverance; and perseverance, character; and character, hope. Now hope does not disappoint, because the love of God has been poured out in our hearts by the Holy Spirit who was given to us.*
> *Romans 5: 3-5*

****

Thanksgiving and Joy

At the writing of this book, Rebecca is thirteen years old, and Andrew is sixteen years old. Just think how much character will have been built in me by the time they are out of their teens!

After I completed all chemotherapy and radiation therapy, Dr. Mitchell started me on Tamoxifen (Nolvadex). It is supposed to help in reducing the recurrence of cancer. I will have to be on it for five years. The chemotherapy put me into early menopause, as Dr. Mitchell had warned it might. Soon, I began having hot flashes. Tamoxifen can also cause hot flashes, so I was getting a double dose of hot flashes, it seemed.

I don't like breaking a sweat just any old time. Neither do I like disturbing my husband by wanting to run the fan all the time, or by throwing the covers back, and a few minutes later, pulling them up again. Even though the hot flashes and sweats are uncomfortable, menopause is one consequence of chemotherapy I can live with. I figure it was going to happen in a few years anyway.

My next three-month check-up was scheduled for February of 1997. I was driving down the road one day, when I suddenly remembered that I was supposed to go see Dr. Mitchell in early February.

It was already February the fifth. So, I stopped by the oncology office to find out if I had already missed my appointment, or if it was scheduled for later. I was told the appointment had been scheduled for earlier that day, and they wondered why I hadn't come. I told them I had forgotten.

I apologized for not having been there at the appointed time, but asked if I could be seen by the doctor while I was there. The receptionist told me Dr. Mitchell was at the other office that afternoon. She did tell me Dr. Gray could see me shortly, however. Dr. Gray had never seen me before, because he had recently joined the practice. He teased that I <u>must</u> be getting better to have forgotten my appointment. I hadn't thought about that before, but he was right. I had other things on my mind now besides cancer and doctor's visits. Things were definitely getting back to normal!

Dr. Gray examined me and found an area in my right breast that caused him some concern. I had thought the area was scar tissue, and had not worried about it. Dr. Gray wanted me to come back in a couple of weeks and let my usual doctor examine me. Since Dr. Mitchell had examined me before, he would probably know if this area had been questionable before.

This was the first thing out of the ordinary that had been found since I had completed therapy. I began to get concerned.

Thanksgiving and Joy

****

For God has not given us a spirit of fear, but of power and of love and of a sound mind.
  II Timothy 1: 7

****

Of course, I shared this news with my base of support. People in my Sunday School class, church, family, and friends were all praying for me. No one, myself included, wanted me to go through cancer again.

Finally the two weeks were up and it was time for my appointment. Dr. Mitchell examined me, and he believed the area was only scar tissue. He assured me if he honestly felt like the area was anything else, he would send me for a mammogram and an ultrasound in a heartbeat. Also, my bloodwork didn't indicate there was any disease process going on in my body. Dr. Gray had not had the benefit of my labwork since my blood had been drawn after Dr. Gray had examined me. I am due to go back in May, and that area will be rechecked. Meanwhile, I am keeping check on it myself.

As I said before, lots of people had been praying for me about this questionable area. Many people came to me after I had the appointment and wanted to know the outcome. They all rejoiced with me when I told them the doctor really believed the area was just scar tissue. Some people cried tears of joy with me when I shared the news. It meant so much to me, knowing so many people were concerned about me. I appreciated everyone's concern.

****

If you abide in Me, and My words abide in you, you will ask what you desire, and it shall be done for you.
John 15: 7

****

I praise God for the faithful prayers of those prayer warriors. God heard their prayers and mine and healed me. I never failed to thank God for the support DeLane and I received during my illness.

Some people asked if I had gone to any cancer support groups. I told them I had never felt the need to go, because I had such a broad base of support, already. These gentle people reminded me support groups are intended not only for support to

Thanksgiving and Joy

be derived from others, but for support to be rendered to others, as well. Now why hadn't I thought of that?

I considered going to support groups, but my schedule was so busy, I didn't know when I would find the time to go. I knew from experience my success story could be used to uplift others. At least, that is what occurred when I related my story to people in the past year and a half. To my surprise, I even thought of writing a book to offer support and encouragement to those who may be confronting breast cancer or some other illness or trial. I knew a book could reach a much greater population than I could reach in a small, support group. But, the thought of writing a book scared me to death. I knew the thought had not been my own thought, so it must have been from God. If God was telling me to do this, I knew I would have to obey, and that is why I was scared. There would be no getting out of it.

Resigned to the possibility of writing a book, I prayed, "Lord, if You want me to write a book to try to encourage other people, You will have to give me the words to say." The only thing I knew how to do was simply tell my story, as I had been doing all along. But, to write a book, and make it interesting, would require God's divine intervention. After all, I'm a person who struggled to write theme papers in school.

When I first had the notion of penning a book, I was working in my second nursing home. My schedule was very hectic and my husband knew it. Upon sharing with DeLane that I was considering writing a book, he laughed and asked, "When are you going to do it? On your days off?" He had a good point. When <u>was</u> I going to find time to write a book? I was confident if God was in it, He would open up the time.

That may also be why I am no longer working in the nursing homes. The private duty work that I do is mostly at night. The night shift has always been the shift I prefer. I suppose it's good not all of us nurses want to work the day or evening shift. If that were the case, there would be a lot of unhappy nurses, because sick people require care twenty-four hours a day.

At any rate, as a private duty nurse, I only have one patient to care for during my shift. Once I have completed my tasks, and the patient has gone to sleep, I often have time to read or write (or do arithmetic - just kidding). Then when my patient requires something else, I get up and meet those needs. I make the most of those free times. It was during those free times, when I started writing a rough draft of this book.

Thanksgiving and Joy

I began writing poems, as well. I had seen an article in a magazine about a poetry-writing contest, and I decided to try to write a poem to enter into the competition. I had written three poems in my life, before that time. I wondered what the subject of this poem could be. Then, I felt impressed to write about how God had blessed me during my illness. When I finished writing the poem, I realized it was twenty-four lines long. To enter the contest, the poem had to be twenty lines or less.

I read back over the poem to see which lines I could leave out. I decided I couldn't delete any of them. The poem told my whole story. I titled it "My God Shall Supply". I also decided to use it on the back of the book cover to explain what my book is about. I finally decided I would have to write another poem to send into the contest, because I just couldn't alter the poem about God's provision.

I was reluctant to tell too many people I was trying to write a book. I guess I didn't want to feel like a failure, if the book never came to fruition. I knew the few people I did tell, were praying for me as I wrote.

I was fairly pleased with the beginning of the book. But, the middle and end left a lot to be desired. It sounded very boggy, and I couldn't think of how to fix it. Since I didn't know how to correct what was wrong, I did the next best thing. I ignored the book, and didn't write for about two months.

One day, at church, I shared with a dear Christian about the report of my mammogram and other tests. She said, "Oh, Glenda, that's wonderful! I will put that as a praise beside of your name in my prayer journal. And, how is the book coming along?"

When Lynne asked that, I knew she had been praying all of this time about the book. I felt like I had somehow let her and God down. God used that incident, to prod me into re-reading the rough draft to see how I might make it sound better. To my amazement, the words started flowing. I praise God for opening up that "writer's block".

Remember my telling God that He would have to give me the words to say in the book? Well, I believe God helped me to write this book. As I sat at the computer and entered the hand-written text, I read back over what I had entered. Quite often, sentences I had written didn't sound exactly right, and I rewrote those parts in a different way. It seemed as if the Holy Spirit was directing me in editing the text. Each time that happened, I stopped and praised God. "Thank you, Lord! That sounds so much better."

Thanksgiving and Joy

****

I will bless the Lord at all times; His praise shall continually be in my mouth.
Psalm 34: 1

****

Since Philippians 4:19 had played such a prominent role in my life, and in the book I was writing, I wanted to personally thank the people who displayed that scripture passage on their license tag. Through several different avenues, I was able to find and meet the owners of that license tag.

Their names are Roger and Linda Byrd, and they are precious Christians. Roger is a minister who is currently serving as interim pastor at a church in Concord, North Carolina.

On March 5, 1997, I drove up to their house. Linda was watering the flowers in front of her house. I parked on the street, went over, and introduced myself to her. I explained I had been wanting to meet her for a year and a half.

She had a puzzled look on her face as I related the story about the tumor being suspicious, and seeing her license tag on the very night I received the news from the surgeon the tumor might be cancerous. As soon as I got to the part about how God had used their license tag and Philippians 4:19 to bless me in such a mighty way, Linda threw her hands up in the air, and started crying, "Oh thank You, Jesus! Thank You, Jesus!"

We were both hugging, and crying, and praising God when her husband, Roger, drove up. Linda yelled, "Roger, come here. You've got to hear this!" We started walking toward him. Then, I noticed the license tag on their car, again, after all this time. It brought that night, immediately into my mind, afresh. I started blubbering all over again. Linda understood, and held me as we wept together.

Roger reached us at about that time. He knew nothing of what had transpired, and he didn't know me. He only knew that I was sobbing for some reason. He said, "Come here, Sister, and let me give you a hug." Roger, Linda, and I had a group hug at that moment. Then we went into their home, where I related my story to them in more detail.

They shared with me how they had come to choose that particular passage, and how they prayed God would use it to bless others. They were thrilled God had used that scripture passage to bless and assure me in such a mighty way. I thanked God that He allowed me to meet these two,

Thanksgiving and Joy

after all this time. I had been praising God for them for a year and a half, and they didn't even know it. Also, their license tag and Philippians 4:19, has been ministering to others with whom I've shared my story over this past year and a half. They were unaware of that, too. We never know how we impact others. Our lives may affect people in a positive or a negative way. I pray my life will be a positive influence on others.

Linda shared with me the route they take to get to church three or four times a week. Would you believe they have been passing within a mile of my house for the past year and a half, and I have never seen that license tag again, until that day?

I made pictures of Roger and Linda, and of the license tag. I had decided I wanted the license tag to be on the front cover of the book . I had planned to draw it on there, but now I would be able to have the picture of the actual license tag on the front cover.

I completed the book in April of 1997, and have been trying to get the book published since then. I have found that not many people want to publish a first-time author. Also, I needed to make some revisions as suggested by Jane Williford, a distant cousin of mine. I do believe God helped me to write the book and wants it to be used to encourage others. Therefore, I have decided to self-publish the book if I don't find a publisher who wants to publish it first.

It has been over 3 years since I found out I had cancer. I am now cancer-free, praise God! Many things have happened since I completed this book in April of 1997. My dad died of bone cancer in October of 1997, and we miss him very much. I am thankful he was able to read my manuscript before he died. He cried when he read it, and felt very sure that the book would be published and would be an encouragement to many other people. Rebecca is now fifteen years old, Andrew is now eighteen years old, and DeLane is older than dirt (just kidding). I no longer have the joint problems or stiffness. My mom has moved closer to me and my sister and our families. My husband and I have remained in our jobs. My hair is almost half way down my back now. Roger and Linda Byrd are no longer the <u>interim</u>, but <u>full-time</u> ministers at First Advent Christian Church in Concord. My husband, children and I still have that strong support base of family, friends, neighbors, and church family. But most of all, God has remained faithful to us during all of those years. I thank Him and praise Him for supplying all of our need just as Philipians 4:19 proclaims.

Thanksgiving and Joy

No.....seeing that license tag and verse on that particular night in 1995, was no coincidence. God put that car beside me at just the right time. His timing is perfect! God promised He would supply all of my needs. He has and still is faithfully keeping His promise. I can't praise Him or thank Him enough for what He has done for me.

Because of God's assurance through Philippians 4:19, I had such a positive outlook during the course of the cancer. I believe having a good attitude about an illness or trial is half of the battle. With a positive attitude, you are more apt to do well. My prayer is that God will use this book to stir you, and help you have a more positive attitude about any trial <u>you</u> may be facing, as well.

All of my praise goes to God, because He is my Creator, Savior, Healer, and Provider. I give Him honor and glory for blessing me with.....<u>Victory Through Breast Cancer.</u>

****

But thanks be to God, who gives us the victory through our Lord Jesus Christ.
I Corinthians 15: 57

Bibliography

American Cancer Society, Breast Cancer Facts and Figures 1996, Atlanta, American Cancer Society, 1995.

_____, The American Cancer Society's Breast Cancer Research Program, Atlanta, American Cancer Society, 1994.

_____, Two Programs, One Purpose: Helping Women With Breast Cancer, Atlanta, American Cancer Society, 1996.

Precious Bible Promises, Nashville, Thomas Nelson, 1983.

Strack, Dr. Jay, editor, The Transformer (New King James Version), Nashville, Thomas Nelson, 1991.

Willmington, Dr. H. L., Willmington's Guide to the Bible, Wheaton, Tyndale House, 1984.

My God Shall Supply

"You have a suspicious tumor,"
   I heard the doctor say.
"This surely can't be true, Doctor!
   Absolutely not! No way!"

What if this is cancer?
   Will I die? What will become of me?
Lord, please give me an answer,
   To comfort me and my family.

That night I received a message:
   PHI 4:19.
It was a scripture passage
   On the license tag I had seen.

My Bible open, I read the verse,
   Tears of joy, I began to cry.
No need to fret or fear the worst,
   All your need, my God shall supply.

Surgery, chemotherapy, radiation,
   And still able to work all week.
Daily I received confirmation,
   That God's promise, always, He does keep.

At year's end, all tests revealed,
  Without a doubt, I'm cancer-free.
Thanksgiving and joy cannot be concealed,
  For the blessings God bestowed upon me.

ORDER FORM

If you would like to order one or more books to share with family, friends, or someone you know who has cancer or is facing a trial, you may do so by using this form.

Name:_____
Address:_____
City:_____
State:_____
Zip:_____

Prices:
- 1 book — $10.95 per book
- 2-5 books — $ 9.95 per book
- 6-10 books — $ 8.95 per book
- 11-15 books — $ 7.95 per book
- 16 or more books — $ 6.95 per book

Sales Tax: Please add 6% for books shipped within North Carolina.

Shipping: # of books being ordered_____. Please include $2.95 shipping for the first book, and $.50 for each additional book.

Payment to: Sumerel Enterprises
( )check   ( )money order   ( )cashier check

Mail Payment to: Sumerel Enterprises
              P.O. Box 905
              Harrisburg, NC 28075-0905

NOTES

NOTES